Electronic Fetal Monitoring (C-EFM®) Certification Review

Antay L. Waters, DNP, APRN, CNM, WHNP-BC, CNRFA, C-EFM, is an assistant professor of nursing at East Texas Baptist University and a practicing board-certified certified nurse midwife and women's health nurse practitioner with the OB Hospitalist Group at CHRISTUS St. Michael in Texarkana, Texas.

Dr. Waters's nursing career began in 2011 as a cardiovascular intensive care nurse, followed by nearly a decade in the operating room and postanesthesia care unit. She is also a certified perioperative nurse (CNOR). In June 2023, she joined the OB Hospitalist Group as an OB hospitalist at CHRISTUS St. Michael in Texarkana, Texas, following over 4 years on staff with Acclaim Physician Group as an OB ED provider at John Peter Smith Hospital in Fort Worth. She is also a certified registered nurse first assist (CRNFA), specializing in obstetric and gynecologic surgery as well as gynecologic robotic surgery.

Dr. Waters is actively involved in multiple professional organizations where she volunteers her time and expertise, including as a content and item writer for the National Certification Corporation for the WHNP exam and the Competency & Credentialing Institute for the CNOR exam. She also continues to mentor DNP and MSN students. Her passion for education has allowed her the opportunity to affect the lives and future careers of baccalaureate nursing students, advanced practice nursing students, medical students, and medical residents. She has presented and published on a variety of topics ranging from obstetric complications, to postoperative pain management, to cardiovascular health, to healthcare risk management through error reduction. She is also serves with the National Association of Nurse Practitioners in Women's Health (NPWH) on the 2023 WHNP Competency Task Force.

Dr. Waters is a legacy member of Texas Nurse Practitioners and a lifetime member of the Association of periOperative Nurses (AORN), as well as the founding president of the Piney Woods Advanced Practice Nurses Association. She is also an active member of the NPWH, American College of Obstetrician and Gynecologists (ACOG), Society of Maternal-Fetal Medicine (SMFM), American College of Nurse Midwives (ACNM), and Sigma Theta Tau International, as well as multiple other professional nursing organizations. She currently resides in Longview, Texas, with her husband, Wes, an inpatient pharmacist at a local hospital, and her 19-year-old daughter, Peyton, a sophomore at East Texas Baptist University studying pre-law Dr. Waters enjoys playing the piano and violin, watching movies, going to plays and concerts, reading, traveling the world, and spending time with family and friends.

Contributor

Shannon Riley DaSilva, DNP, APRN, CNM, John Peter Smith Hospital Health Network, Fort Worth, Texas; Baylor University, Louise Herrington School of Nursing, Dallas, Texas, contributed Chapters 4 and 5.

Electronic Fetal Monitoring (C-EFM®) Certification Review

Antay L. Waters, DNP, APRN, CNM, WHNP-BC, CNRFA, C-EFM

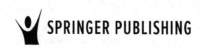
SPRINGER PUBLISHING

Springer Publishing Company, LLC
www.springerpub.com

Acquisitions Editor: Jaclyn Koshofer
Compositor: Transforma

ISBN: 978-0-8261-9301-8
ebook ISBN: 978-0-8261-9302-5
DOI: 10.1891/9780826193025

24 25 26 27 / 5 4 3 2 1

The author and the publisher of this Work have made every effort to use sources believed to be reliable to provide information that is accurate and compatible with the standards generally accepted at the time of publication. The author and publisher shall not be liable for any special, consequential, or exemplary damages resulting, in whole or in part, from the readers' use of, or reliance on, the information contained in this book. The publisher has no responsibility for the persistence or accuracy of URLs for external or third-party Internet websites referred to in this publication and does not guarantee that any content on such websites is, or will remain, accurate or appropriate.

Library of Congress Cataloging-in-Publication Data

Names: Waters, Antay L., author. | DaSilva, Shannon Riley, author.
Title: Electronic fetal monitoring (C-EFM) certification review / Antay L.
  Waters ; contributor, Shannon Riley DaSilva.
Description: New York : Springer Publishing Company, [2024] | Includes
  bibliographical references and index.
Identifiers: LCCN 2023037239 | ISBN 9780826193018 (paperback) | ISBN
  9780826193025 (ebook)
Subjects: MESH: Cardiotocography | Prenatal Diagnosis | Study Guide
Classification: LCC RG628 | NLM WQ 18.2 | DDC
  618.3/2075076–dc23/eng/20230921
LC record available at https://lccn.loc.gov/2023037239

Contact sales@springerpub.com to receive discount rates on bulk purchases.

Publisher's Note: **New and used products purchased from third-party sellers are not guaranteed for quality, authenticity, or access to any included digital components.**

Printed in the United States of America by Gasch Printing.

C-EFM® is a registered trademark of the National Certification Corporation (NCC). NCC does not sponsor nor endorse this resource, nor does it have a proprietary relationship with Springer Publishing.

This book is dedicated to my current and former students and colleagues, who have made me a better educator and clinician. Your tireless efforts have allowed our profession to grow and improve for our patients and society. I am inspired by your commitment, compassion, and perseverance to the nursing profession regardless of the circumstances and challenges.

Contents

Reviewers

Reveca Alaniz, MSN, RNC-OB, RN Outreach and Clinical Educator for Women and Infants, John Peter Smith Health Network, Fort Worth, Texas

Shannon Riley DaSilva, DNP, APRN, CNM, John Peter Smith Hospital Health Network, Fort Worth, Texas; Baylor University, Louise Herrington School of Nursing, Dallas, Texas

Amy Decker, MSN, RNC-OB, C-EFM, Clinical Educator, Women's Services, John Peter Smith Health Network, Fort Worth, Texas

Peggy Rhodes, BSN, RNC-EFM, Staff RN, Obstetrics Triage, John Peter Smith Hospital Health Network, Fort Worth, Texas

Samantha Skinner, MSN, RNC-OB, C-EFM, Aya Healthcare, San Diego, California

Preface

Welcome to the first edition of *Electronic Fetal Monitoring C-EFM® Certification Review*. This book was created to serve all clinicians caring for obstetric patients undergoing electronic fetal monitoring (EFM) for any indication in order to provide consistent, evidence-based care and reduce inconsistencies in practice. This book presents material and practice questions based on the National Certification Corporation's (NCC) Certification in Electronic Fetal Monitoring (C-EFM®) exam blueprint in a succinct, direct, easy-to-read and -understand manner. The practice questions were written and reviewed by practicing clinicians holding the C-EFM credential.

This book can also be used to support student education during any educational program covering fetal monitoring, including baccalaureate and graduate nursing and medical students. Students can use this book to enhance study habits, review for academic exams, improve test-taking skills, reinforce knowledge, and avoid test-taking errors. Faculty can use this book and practice questions throughout their curriculum by integrating them into polling technology, classroom discussion, case studies, and pre- and post-lecture reviews to evaluate for knowledge gaps.

Electronic Fetal Monitoring C-EFM® Certification Review contains a comprehensive review of foundational knowledge needed by all clinicians providing care to patients undergoing any type of fetal monitoring. Review of advanced pathophysiology, pharmacology, and health assessment provides the underpinning for the rest of the content. These key chapters review both maternal and fetal pathophysiology, fetal oxygenation and acid-base status, potential obstetric complications and associated interventions, and EFM equipment fundamental to successfully passing the exam. The book contains detailed content, case studies, and practice questions covering the topics included on the exam blueprints. Practice questions have specific rationales explaining why the correct answer is correct and the distractors are incorrect. These questions will build and reinforce your knowledge base. A full-scale practice exam that is representative in length, variety, and complexity of the C-EFM exam is provided and can be taken in a timed format to assess your abilities under pressure.

Antay Waters

Acknowledgments

This book could not have been possible without my expert contributor and reviewers. Your expertise will assist women's health clinicians to pursue the next level of certification in order to provide exceptional, evidence-based care for women during one of the most vulnerable times of life.

I would like to extend sincerest gratitude to all my colleagues at East Texas Baptist University, Acclaim Multi-Specialty Group, and JPS Health Network for providing support and encouragement throughout this process. Drs. Kevin and Melissa Reeves—even though you often had no idea what I was talking about, you always supported and encouraged me to follow my dreams and provided valuable insight throughout this process.

I would also like to specifically thank a few colleagues in particular who have provided unwavering support and encouragement throughout not only this process but also throughout my career as a nurse, women's health nurse practitioner, and certified nurse midwife. Dr. Chuck Safely—you propelled my career forward in unimaginable ways, always encouraging me to follow my dreams despite the odds. You spurred my love for women's health that brought me to where I am today. Drs. Tracy Papa and Becky Reyes—you have been among the greatest supporters in my life, both personally and professionally. Your wisdom allowed me the opportunity to provide excellent, evidence-based care for countless women in Tarrant County with confidence and now to share that knowledge through this work. To my fellow CNM colleague and friend, Arnette Kelley—you remind me to never give up, even when the odds seem insurmountable. Your encouragement has taken me places I never dreamed possible! I am so thankful for each of you!

Thank you to Jaclyn Koshofer and Jennifer Ehlers at Springer Publishing Company for providing the opportunity to publish this book. I sincerely appreciate the faith you've had in me, your guidance through the process, and unwavering support despite setbacks. You have been essential to making this project come to fruition. It has been an absolute pleasure to work with you!

Pass Guarantee

If you use this resource to prepare for your exam and do not pass, you may return it for a refund of your full purchase price, excluding tax, shipping, and handling. To receive a refund, return your product along with a copy of your exam score report and original receipt showing purchase of new product (not used). Product must be returned and received within 180 days of the original purchase date. Refunds will be issued within 8 weeks from acceptance and approval. One offer per person and address. This offer is valid for U.S. residents only. Void where prohibited. To initiate a refund, please contact Customer Service at csexamprep@springerpub.com.

Introduction to the Electronic Fetal Monitoring Exam

Antay L. Waters

▶ INTRODUCTION

Through certification, nurses and other healthcare professionals validate their expert knowledge in a given practice area. While state licensure exams through the National Council of State Boards of Nursing (NCSBN) verify that an entry-level nurse is ready for practice, specialty certification confirms "the ability of expert nurses to provide evidence-based care at all levels of acuity in a specialized area" (Martin et al., 2015).

The goal of this review book is to provide a comprehensive and up-to-date review of electronic fetal monitoring based on the content outline of the National Certification Corporation (NCC) Certification in Electronic Fetal Monitoring (C-EFM®) exam in order to promote certification exam success and enhance clinical practice.

▶ OBJECTIVES

- Discuss the importance of obtaining specialty certification as well as the role of specialty C-EFM®.
- Review exam eligibility and scoring for the NCC C-EFM® exam.
- Review exam content and testing methods employed for the NCC C-EFM® exam.

▶ KEY TERMS

- **Certification in Electronic Fetal Monitoring (C-EFM®) Examination:** The certification exam administered by the NCC that tests expert knowledge and proficiency in the examination and interpretation of electronic fetal monitoring in the clinical setting
- **National Certification Corporation (NCC):** An organization that provides national certification programs for nurses, physicians, advanced practice nurses, and other licensed healthcare professionals
- **Professional Certification:** A third-party designation granted by an authority in the field and earned by an individual, attesting to that individual's proficiency, knowledge, and qualification to care for a specific patient population or subset of patients

▶ PURPOSE OF PROFESSIONAL CERTIFICATION

Why obtain professional certification? Professional certification demonstrates to the public and the professional healthcare community a mastery of specialized knowledge by meeting psychometric requirements through examination (Barbé & Kimble, 2018). It also demonstrates a commitment to lifelong learning and excellence, including remaining up to date on changing practices and technology (Junger et al., 2016). Specialty certification, "when fully realized, has the potential to improve patient outcomes, contribute to patient safety goals, and elevate [the] profession" (Stobinski, 2019). The 2010 Institute of Medicine report *The Future of Nursing: Leading Change, Advancing Health* argues that lifelong learning is necessary for continued competence when providing care for changing and diverse patient groups.

ABOUT THE NATIONAL CERTIFICATION CORPORATION

Since its inception in 1975, NCC has awarded more than 195,000 certifications to licensed healthcare professionals including nurses, physicians, advanced practice providers, and others. Nursing and advanced practice nursing certifications may be awarded in obstetric, gynecologic, and neonatal specialties, while multidisciplinary certifications are available for electronic fetal monitoring, neonatal pediatric transport, obstetric and neonatal quality and safety, care of the extremely low birth weight neonate, and neonatal neuro-intensive care. While the NCC credential holds no licensing authority, high standards are reflected in the certification process.

▶ THE NATIONAL CERTIFICATION CORPORATION C-EFM® EXAMINATION

The NCC C-EFM® exam consists of 125 questions: 100 scored questions and 25 pretest questions that do not count toward the final result. There is no indication in the exam as to which items are scored versus which are pretest. Candidates have 2 hours to complete the exam. NCC uses a single-question format for all exams. Each question contains a premise (stem) and three answer choices. The answer choices are alphabetized based on the first word of the answer choice to randomize answers. Questions test basic knowledge as well as application, analysis, and evaluation of information. Any items that contain laboratory values will show results in conventional units with international units in parentheses. Medications will include both generic and trade names where appropriate (NCC, 2022a).

ELIGIBILITY

To be eligible to sit for the NCC C-EFM® exam, candidates must hold a current, active, unencumbered license in the United States or Canada as a physician, registered nurse, nurse practitioner, nurse midwife or midwife, physician assistant, or paramedic. A copy of the applicable license, including name, license number, licensing state or province, type of license, and expiration date, must be submitted to NCC before receiving an authorization to test.

Following submission of the application, it will be reviewed by NCC to determine qualification and eligibility to test, which may take up to 2 weeks. Once the application is approved, an examination eligibility letter is sent via email. Candidates must schedule their exam within the first 30 days of the eligibility window to occur within 90 days.

MAINTENANCE OF NATIONAL CERTIFICATION CORPORATION C-EFM® CERTIFICATION

Certifications are approved to meet the American Board of Obstetrics and Gynecology (ABOG) Part IV credit as an ABOG-approved Simulation Course for Maintenance of Certification (MOC). Part IV credit may be earned in the year of initial certification as well as for certification maintenance (NCC, 2022b).

SCORING

All NCC examinations are criterion references, meaning the passing score is based on predetermined criteria established by the NCC board of directors. NCC uses item response theory, or Rasch analysis, for exam analysis. Item response theory is the study of tests and exam scores based on assumptions involving the mathematical relationship between item responses and ability. Each item is assigned a difficulty and an ability level. The higher the difficulty level, the higher the assigned ability score. A passing score is determined based on the number of questions answered correctly. The ability score increases for each question answered correctly and decreases for each question answered incorrectly. As there are multiple exam forms in use, equating is used to convert all results to a common scale because the difficulty of the exam determines the actual number of questions that must be answered correctly in order to achieve a passing score. Therefore, someone who receives a more difficult exam will need to answer fewer questions correctly than someone who receives an easier form of the exam. Test result reports will identify pass/fail status and give feedback on each individual content area in the form of the following descriptors: very weak, weak, average, strong, and very strong (NCC, 2022a).

CONTENT OUTLINE

The NCC C-EFM® exam consists of five key areas: electronic fetal monitoring, physiology, pattern recognition and intervention, fetal assessment methods, and professional issues. The major focus is on pattern recognition and intervention; however, this does not mean candidates will simply have to interpret electronic fetal monitoring strips. Candidates must be able to read a clinical scenario and understand what is happening beyond the visual representation on the electronic fetal monitoring strip.

Electronic Monitoring Equipment (5%)

Potential questions related to electronic fetal monitoring equipment may include:

- External and internal monitoring equipment, indications, and contraindications for use
- Identification of artifact
- Identification and correction of signal ambiguity
- Electronic fetal monitoring equipment failure and troubleshooting (NCC, 2022a)

Physiology (11%)

Potential questions related to uteroplacental physiology may include:

- Uteroplacental circulation
- Fetal circulation
- Fetal heart regulation
- Factors affecting fetal oxygenation, including uterine activity, maternal factors, anesthesia, medications, placental factors, umbilical blood flow, and acid-base and cord blood gases (NCC, 2022a)

Pattern Recognition and Intervention (70%)

Potential questions related to pattern recognition and intervention may include:

- Recognition of fetal heart rate baseline (bradycardia, tachycardia, variability, and sinusoidal)
- Identification of fetal heart rate variability and potential causes of abnormal variability
- Recognition of abnormal uterine activity related to complications (decreased uterine blood flow, hypertonic uterine dysfunction, and tachysystole)
- Identification of fetal dysrhythmias (supraventricular tachycardia, congenital heart block, and ectopic beats)
- Synthesis of implications of maternal complications (preterm labor, hypertension, post-term/post-date pregnancy, diabetes, multiple gestations, infections, and maternal obesity)
- Understanding of uteroplacental complications (placenta previa, placental abruption, and uterine rupture/scar dehiscence)
- Fetal complications (traumatic injury, cord compression, hypoxemia, and demise)
- Fetal heart rate accelerations and decelerations (early, variable, late, and prolonged)
- Normal uterine activity (resting tone, contraction frequency, contraction duration, and contraction intensity; NCC, 2022a)

Fetal Assessment Methods (9%)

Potential questions related to fetal assessment methods may include:

- Various auscultation methods
- Assessment of fetal movement and appropriate use and methods of fetal stimulation
- Indications and implications for fetal nonstress testing
- Indications and implications for fetal biophysical profile
- Analysis and interpretation of fetal cord blood and acid-base balance (NCC, 2022a)

Professional Issues (5%)

Potential questions related to professional issues may include:

- Legal and ethical issues
- Patient safety
- Quality improvement (NCC, 2022a)

> **Clinical Pearl**
>
> Do not rely solely on ability to visually interpret electronic fetal monitoring strips, despite pattern recognition and intervention being the largest portion of the exam. This section of the exam also encompasses the understanding of maternal, fetal, and uteroplacental complications when relayed in a written clinical scenario.

ASSOCIATED COMPETENCIES

In addition to the previously mentioned content areas, 10 associated competencies are addressed by the NCC C-EFM® exam, including:

- Apply knowledge of maternal-fetal assessment methods when selecting electronic fetal monitoring or intermittent auscultation to evaluate fetal status
- Interpret data from the electronic fetal monitor to differentiate between actual fetal data and equipment failure
- Use knowledge of the advantages and disadvantages of electronic fetal monitoring to provide information to the pregnant patient and their support person(s)
- Apply knowledge of fetal heart rate regulation to the interpretation of electronic fetal monitoring data
- Identify and interpret significance of fetal heart rate patterns
- Interpret data from electronic fetal monitoring to differentiate between normal and abnormal fetal heart rate patterns
- Apply knowledge of common pregnancy complications to the development of a comprehensive plan of care based on electronic fetal monitoring data
- Apply knowledge of uteroplacental and maternal-fetal physiology as related to fetal oxygenation
- Identify indications of adjunct fetal assessment, and incorporate findings into the plan of care
- Incorporate knowledge of current practice and legal practices into nursing care (NCC, 2022a)

▶ FETAL MONITORING: A HISTORICAL PERSPECTIVE

Fetal heart rate assessment is an indirect measure of fetal oxygenation during the antepartum and intrapartum periods. The evolution of fetal heart rate monitoring was shaped by clinicians and researchers with a desire to decrease fetal morbidity and mortality, beginning with unassisted auscultation and palpation techniques. The technologies and techniques in use today are the result of more than a century of research and development by those committed to improving birth outcomes through the identification and implementation of best practice for fetal heart rate assessment, interpretation, intervention, and evaluation.

EARLY DEVELOPMENT

More than 350 years ago, French physician Marsac described fetal heart sounds; however, it took another 150 years before fetal heart tone auscultation became routine practice in western Europe and North America (Gultekin-Zootzmann, 1975). The use of electronic fetal monitoring is a much more recent event, entering the scene in the 1950s and 1960s, with the first commercial fetal monitor becoming available in 1968 (Freeman & Garite, 1981). During this time, the rise of electronics was at its peak. While electronic fetal monitoring is the term used in the western world, the term used in other parts of the world is cardiotocography, or CTG, from the Greek words *kardia*, meaning heart, and *tokos*, meaning labor and childbirth. While electronic fetal monitoring technology has made vast strides over the last 60 years, the goal of improving safety and outcomes has not wavered.

PRESENT-DAY ELECTRONIC FETAL MONITORING

In Ayres-de-Campos and Arulkumaran (2015), the International Federation of Gynecology and Obstetrics promoted the largest consensus to date on intrapartum fetal monitoring with the objective of standardizing terminology, interpretation, and clinical management. Today, electronic fetal monitoring is used in the vast majority of births in almost every type of birth setting, from use of handheld Dopplers for intermittent monitoring to use of larger machines for continuous fetal monitoring.

ADJUNCT SURVEILLANCE METHODS

Electronic fetal monitoring was originally intended to be used as a screening tool to detect fetal compromise early enough to intervene and prevent adverse neurological outcomes or death secondary to asphyxia or oxygen deprivation. The utility of a tool such as this is directly related to its sensitivity, specificity, reliability, and validity.

A normal/category I electronic fetal monitoring tracing correctly identifies an oxygenated fetus with a high level of sensitivity and is unlikely to have false-negative interpretations. When a category I tracing is present, clinicians typically agree that the fetus is well-oxygenated. When an indeterminate/category II tracing is present, there is a low level of specificity, including the possibility of a false-positive or false-negative interpretation. Since these are not necessarily predictive of abnormal acid-base status, clinicians may have differing opinions and interpretations. While category III tracings have a low positive predictive value, a general consensus exists that the risk of fetal acidemia is high enough to warrant intervention despite the low positive predictive value.

Adjunct methods have been developed to complement fetal monitoring and provide additional information related to fetal oxygenation status. Fetal assessment late in pregnancy hastened a new field of care: antepartum fetal surveillance, leading to the development of specialized antepartum testing centers and a new obstetric subspecialty—maternal-fetal medicine (Resnik et al., 2019).

▶ TEST-TAKING STRATEGIES

There is no best way to prepare for an exam because learning is an ongoing process, including self-discovery. Each candidate is the best person to determine the best way to prepare for their certification exam.

COMMON TEST-TAKING STRATEGIES

Some common exam strategies that are applicable to the NCC C-EFM® exam include:

- Get a good night's rest the night before, and eat a healthy breakfast the morning of the exam.
- Arrive at the testing center on time, or even a few minutes early.
- Know where to go ahead of time. This will help alleviate potential stress the morning of the exam. If possible, drive to the testing site prior to exam day.
- Read each question in its entirety, watching for words like *is, is not, always,* or *sometimes.* Do not stop halfway through a question and assume what is being asked.
- Think of the answer to the question before reading the answer choices. This may lead to the correct answer.
- Learn to identify and ignore distractors. They are there to do exactly that—distract.
- Eliminate obviously incorrect answers first, and then consider the remaining options.
- Be aware of time spent on each question. Do not spend too much time on one question. Instead, flag it and come back to it.
- Answer every question even if unsure if the answer is correct. There is no penalty for incorrect answers.

Clinical Pearl

Use of test-taking strategies allows for decreased stress and anxiety for the candidate, improving overall likelihood of success.

▶ KEY POINTS

- Professional certification demonstrates to the public and the professional healthcare community a mastery of specialized knowledge by meeting psychometric requirements through examination.
- Understanding the content outline for the NCC C-EFM® exam is imperative to set oneself up for success.
- Using effective test-taking strategies will allow the candidate to be better prepared for the NCC C-EFM® exam.

▶ REFERENCES

Ayres-de-Campos, D., & Arulkumaran, S. (2015). FIGO intrapartum fetal monitoring expert consensus panel FIGO consensus guidelines on intrapartum fetal monitoring: Introduction. *International Journal of Gynecology and Obstetrics*, 131(1), 3–4.

Barbé, T., & Kimble, L. (2018). What is the value of nurse educator certification? A comparison study of certified and noncertified nurse educators. *Nurse Educator Perspective*, 39(2), 66–71.

Committee on the Robert Wood Johnson Foundation Initiative on the Future of Nursing at the Institute of Medicine. (2010). *The future of nursing: Leading change, advancing health*. National Academies Press.

Freeman, R. K., & Garite, T. J. (1981). *Fetal heart rate monitoring*. Williams & Wilkins.

Gultekin-Zootzmann, B. (1975). The history of monitoring the human fetus. *Journal of Perinatal Medicine*, 3(1), 135–144.

Junger, S., Trinkle, N., & Hall, N. (2016). Nurse leader certification preparation: How are confidence levels impacted? *Journal of Nursing Management*, 24, 775–779.

Martin, L., Arenas-Montoya, N., & Barnett, T. (2015). Impact of nurse certification rates on patient satisfaction and outcomes: A literature review. *Journal of Continuing Education in Nursing*, 46(12), 549–554.

National Certification Corporation. (2022a). *2022 Candidate guide: Electronic fetal monitoring*. https://www.nccwebsite.org/content/documents/cms/efm-candidate_guide.pdf

National Certification Corporation. (2022b). *Certification exams: Electronic fetal monitoring*. https://www.nccwebsite.org/certification-exams/details/1/electronic-fetal-monitoring

Resnik, R., Lockwood, C. J., Moore, T. R., Greene, M. F., Copel, J. A., & Silver, R. M. (2019). *Creasy & Resnik's maternal-fetal medicine: Principles and practice*. Elsevier.

Stobinski, J. (2019). CNOR recertification: Why continuing education alone is no longer sufficient. *AORN Journal*, 110(3), 273–281.

Fetal Assessment Methods

Antay L. Waters

2

▶ INTRODUCTION

The ultimate goal of antepartum fetal assessment is to reduce the risk of stillbirth. Fetal assessment methods during both the antepartum and the intrapartum periods are selected based on gestational age, available technology and resources, patient presentation, and pregnancy complications, with the purpose of assessing the adequacy of uteroplacental perfusion at any given time. While currently available fetal assessment methods are effective screening tools for predicting fetal well-being, they are nondiagnostic for fetal hypoxia or acidosis. This chapter focuses on the techniques available for assessing the fetus in utero, including both fetal heart rate (FHR) and uterine activity, as well as their limitations, procedures, and potential troubleshooting tips; the analysis of neonatal umbilical cord blood sampling; and the role of the clinician in the fetal assessment process.

▶ OBJECTIVES

- Discuss indications for antenatal fetal surveillance based on maternal-fetal presentation and pregnancy complications.
- Understand various technologies available for antepartum fetal surveillance as well as indications and contraindications for each.
- Differentiate the appropriate uses of both intermittent and continuous fetal monitoring, including professional society recommendations for each.
- Review limitations and troubleshooting tips for various methods of FHR assessment.
- Analyze fetal umbilical cord sampling as a tool for evaluating neonatal status.

▶ KEY TERMS

- **Artifact:** Inaccurate variation or absence of the FHR on the tracing due to mechanical or technical limitations or electrical interference on the monitoring system
- **Auscultation:** Action of listening to sounds as part of the diagnostic process
- **Base deficit:** Measures the amount of base buffer reserves below normal levels. A large positive base deficit (≥12 mmol/L) indicates that base buffers have been used to buffer base acids, sufficient base buffers are not present, and metabolic acidosis is present
- **Base excess:** Measures the amount of base buffer reserves above normal levels. A large negative base excess (≥−12 mmol/L) indicates that base buffers have been used to buffer base acids, sufficient base buffers are not present, and metabolic acidosis is present
- **Nonstress test:** Common antenatal test used to evaluate fetal oxygenation status, so named because nothing is done to place stress on the fetus during the exam
- **Vibroacoustic stimulation:** Simple, noninvasive technique using a handheld device over the maternal abdomen near the fetal head, emitting sound at a predetermined level for several seconds in an attempt to arouse the fetus and stimulate fetal activity

▶ INDICATIONS FOR ANTEPARTUM FETAL SURVEILLANCE

Given the near-limitless number of possible complications, especially unanticipated, it is impossible to compile a completely comprehensive list of all antenatal conditions for which antepartum fetal surveillance is indicated. The American College of Obstetricians and Gynecologists (ACOG) provides guidance on the initiation of antepartum fetal surveillance for conditions with a frequency of occurrence greater than .8 per 1,000 that are associated with a relative risk for stillbirth of more than twice that of other pregnancies without the same condition (Table 2.1; American College of Obstetricians and Gynecologists [ACOG], 2021). While evidence based, these are only suggestions, rather than requirements. Antepartum fetal surveillance requires individualization based on clinical presentation and maternal-fetal assessment of the clinician.

Table 2.1 Indications for Antepartum Fetal Surveillance[*]

Factor	Suggested Gestational Age to Begin Antenatal Fetal Surveillance	Suggested Frequency of Antenatal Fetal Surveillance
FETAL		
Growth Restriction[1]		
UAD: Normal or with elevated impedance to flow in UA with diastolic flow present; with normal AFI and no other concurrent maternal or fetal conditions	At diagnosis[2]	Once or twice weekly
UAD: AEDV or concurrent conditions (oligohydramnios, maternal comorbidity [e.g., preeclampsia, chronic hypertension])	At diagnosis[2]	Twice weekly[3] or consider inpatient management
UAD REDV	At diagnosis[2]	Inpatient management'
Multiple Gestation		
Twins, uncomplicated dichorionic	36 0/7 weeks	Weekly
Twins, dichorionic, complicated by maternal or fetal disorders, such as fetal growth restriction	At diagnosis[2]	Individualized
Twins, uncomplicated monochorionic-diamniotic	32 0/7 weeks[4]	Weekly
Twins, complicated monochorionic-diamniotic (i.e., TTTS)	Individualized	Individualized
Twins, monoamniotic	Individualized	Individualized
Triplets and higher order multiples	Individualized	Individualized
Decreased fetal movement	At diagnosis[3]	Once[5]
Fetal anomalies and aneuploidy	Individualized	Individualized
MATERNAL		
Hypertension, Chronic		
Controlled with medications	32 0/7 weeks	Weekly
Poorly controlled or with associated medical conditions	At diagnosis[2]	Individualized
Gestational Hypertension/Preeclampsia		
Without severe features	At diagnosis[2,3]	Twice weekly
With severe features	At diagnosis[2,3]	Daily
Diabetes		
Gestational, controlled on medications without other comorbidities	32 0/7 weeks	Once or twice weekly
Gestational, poorly controlled	32 0/7 weeks	Twice weekly
Pregestational	32 0/7 weeks[6]	Twice weekly

(continued)

Table 2.1 Indications for Antepartum Fetal Surveillance* (*continued*)

Factor	Suggested Gestational Age to Begin Antenatal Fetal Surveillance	Suggested Frequency of Antenatal Fetal Surveillance
Systemic Lupus Erythematosus		
Uncomplicated	By 32 0/7 weeks	Weekly
Complicated[7]	At diagnosis[2]	Individualized
Antiphospholipid syndrome	By 32 0/7 weeks[8]	Twice weekly
Sickle Cell Disease		
Uncomplicated	32 0/7 weeks	Once or twice weekly
Complicated[9]	At diagnosis[2]	Individualized
Hemoglobinopathies other than Hb SS disease	Individualized	Individualized
Renal disease (Cr greater than 1.4 mg/dL)	32 0/7 weeks	Once or twice weekly
Thyroid disorders, poorly controlled	Individualized	Individualized
In vitro fertilization	36 0/7 weeks	Weekly
Substance Use		
Alcohol, 5 or more drinks per week	36 0/7 weeks	Weekly
Polysubstance use	Individualized	Individualized
Prepregnancy BMI		
Prepregnancy BMI 35.0–39.9 kg/m²	37 0/7 weeks	Weekly
Prepregnancy BMI 40 kg/m² or above	34 0/7 weeks	Weekly
Maternal age older than 35 years	Individualized[10]	Individualized
OBSTETRIC		
Previous Stillbirth		
At or after 32 0/7 weeks	32 0/7 weeks[11]	Once or twice weekly
Before 32 0/7 weeks' gestation	Individualized	Individualized
History of other adverse pregnancy outcomes in immediately preceding pregnancy		
Previous fetal growth restriction requiring preterm delivery	32 0/7 weeks	Weekly
Previous preeclampsia requiring preterm delivery	32 0/7 weeks	Weekly
Cholestasis	At diagnosis[2]	Once or twice weekly
Late term	41 0/7 weeks	Once or twice weekly
Abnormal Serum Markers[12]		
PAPP-A less than or equal to the fifth percentile (.4 MoM)	36 0/7 weeks	Weekly
Second-trimester inhibin A equal to or greater than 2.0 MoM	36 0/7 weeks	Weekly
PLACENTAL		
Chronic placental abruption[13]	At diagnosis[2]	Once or twice weekly
Vasa previa	Individualized	Individualized
Velamentous cord insertion	36 0/7 weeks	Weekly
Single UA	36 0/7 weeks	Weekly

(*continued*)

Table 2.1 Indications for Antepartum Fetal Surveillance[*] (*continued*)

Factor	Suggested Gestational Age to Begin Antenatal Fetal Surveillance	Suggested Frequency of Antenatal Fetal Surveillance
Isolated oligohydramnios (single deepest vertical pocket less than 2 cm)	At diagnosis[2,3]	Once or twice weekly
Polyhydramnios, moderate to severe (deepest vertical pocket equal to or greater than 12 cm or AFI equal to or greater than 30 cm)	32 0/7 to 34 0/7 weeks[14]	Once or twice weekly

[*]The guidance offered in this table should be construed only as suggestions, not mandates. Ultimately, individualization about if and when to offer antenatal fetal surveillance is advised.
[1]Estimated fetal weight or abdominal circumference less than the 10th percentile.
[2]Or at a gestational age when delivery would be considered because of abnormal test results.
[3]If not delivered.
[4]In addition to routine surveillance for twin-twin transfusion syndrome and other monochorionic twin complications.
[5]Repeat if decreased fetal movement recurs.
[6]Or earlier for poor glycemic control or end-organ damage.
[7]Such as active lupus nephritis, recent lupus flare, antiphospholipid antibodies with prior fetal loss, anti-RO/SSA or anti-La/SSB antibodies, or thrombosis.
[8]Individualize, take into consideration obstetric history, number of positive antibodies, and current pregnancy complications.
[9]Such as maternal hypertension, vaso-occlusive crisis, placental insufficiency, fetal growth restriction.
[10]Based on cumulative risk when present with other factors.
[11]Or starting 1 to 2 weeks before the gestational age of the previous stillbirth.
[12]If serum screening for aneuploidy is performed, the results may be considered in determining whether antenatal fetal surveillance should be performed.
[13]In individuals who are candidates for outpatient management.
[14]Or at diagnosis if diagnosed after 32 0/7 to 34 0/7 weeks.

AEDV, absent end-diastolic velocity; AFI, amniotic fluid index; BMI, body mass index; Cr, creatinine; MoM, multiples of the median; PAPP-A, pregnancy-associated plasma protein A; REDV, reversed end-diastolic flow; TTTS, twin-to-twin transfusion syndrome; UA, umbilical artery; UAD, umbilical artery Doppler.

Source: American College of Obstetrics and Gynecology. (2021). ACOG practice bulletin 229. Antepartum fetal surveillance. *Obstetrics and Gynecology, 137*(6), e116–e127. https://doi.org/10.1097/AOG .0000000000004410

Antepartum fetal surveillance has been categorized based on gestational age–adjusted risk of stillbirth, falling into three categories:

1. At or by 32 weeks and 0 days of gestation
2. At or by 36 weeks and 0 days of gestation
3. At or beyond 39 weeks and 0 days of gestation, if undelivered

While initiating antenatal fetal surveillance at 32 weeks and 0 days of gestation or later is appropriate for most at-risk patients, those with multiple or extremely high-risk conditions should be considered for antenatal fetal surveillance beginning at the gestational age when delivery would be considered for perinatal benefit (ACOG, 2021). Regardless of the timing, shared decision-making between the patient and the clinician is vital, especially when decisions are made near the point of viability when extensive neonatal resuscitation may be required. Patients should be appropriately counseled and be part of the decision-making process to initiate antenatal fetal surveillance, particularly concerning whether intervention or delivery will be considered for nonreassuring fetal status. A multidisciplinary approach should also include neonatology to allow patients and their families to make well-informed decisions for all parties involved. Allowing patient autonomy in this decision is imperative.

Clinical Pearl

While many algorithms exist to determine the need for antenatal fetal surveillance, each case should be evaluated on an individual basis to determine the need for antenatal testing, especially given its noninvasive nature.

▶ ELECTRONIC FETAL MONITORING EQUIPMENT

Electronic fetal monitoring (EFM) is a screening procedure in which monitors are used to continuously record the heart rate of the fetus and the activity of the patient's uterus during the antepartum and intrapartum periods. Continuous EFM is associated with many known medical risks to pregnant patients, without providing any proven benefit to the fetus in low-risk pregnancies (ACOG, 2009; Alfirevic et al., 2006). Continuously monitoring the fetus during labor is associated with a significant increase in Cesarean section, operative vaginal delivery, and maternal infection with no reduction of cerebral palsy or neonatal death when it is compared with intermittent auscultation (IA; Alfirevic et al., 2006). Although neonatal seizures are rare events (1 in 500 births), the incidence is decreased with the use of EFM, but only in the setting of high-risk pregnancies. There is no noted difference in uncomplicated pregnancies (Chen et al., 2011). For every 661 patients who receive continuous EFM during labor, one neonatal seizure will be prevented (Alfirevic et al., 2006).

Although the term used to monitor fetal well-being is *electronic fetal monitoring*, the monitors currently used measure two distinct parameters. The first is the FHR, but equally important is the second: the pattern of uterine activity. FHR may be measured with an external monitoring device or an internal device, known as a fetal scalp electrode. Both of these transmit a signal to a console where the patterns are printed on a graph or transmitted to a video screen running at a rate of 3 cm/min. The display is a two-channel display, where the top channel is the FHR displayed in beats per minute, and the bottom channel is the uterine activity pattern coinciding with the displayed fetal cardiac activity. Uterine activity can also be measured with both external and internal devices. The external option is known as a tocodynamometer, while the internal option is called an intrauterine pressure catheter (IUPC).

EFM machines currently use Doppler signal processing technology, referred to as autocorrelation. Autocorrelation entails the digitization and analysis of the reflection of the ultrasound waveforms to produce the images seen on fetal monitoring tracings. This process is described by Schwartz and Young (2006) as computerized smoothing of waveforms. The internal computer within the fetal monitoring system averages three consecutive beat-to-beat intervals, then assigns the FHR. Autocorrelation works by matching each incoming waveform with the previous one, repetitively analyzing small segments of the waveforms. Important information will have a regular form, while random noises and artifact are discarded.

▶ TECHNIQUES FOR ASSESSMENT OF THE FETAL HEART RATE

Various techniques are available for assessment of the FHR. Choosing the most appropriate method is imperative for accurate results related to fetal status in the current intrauterine environment and indirect assessment of fetal oxygenation. Regardless of which assessment method is chosen, clinicians are responsible for possessing the knowledge required to recognize and respond to the results obtained from fetal assessment methods. Without appropriately trained clinicians, use of EFM only increases the risk to patients.

ABDOMINAL ASSESSMENT

Locating the fetal back for optimal auscultation is the first step in the fetal assessment process. Leopold maneuvers may be performed to identify fetal position and location of the fetal back. Box 2.1 details the steps required for proper Leopold maneuvers. Typically, the FHR is heard best over the fetal back, especially when the fetal back is against the maternal uterine abdominal wall. When a fetus is in an occiput posterior position, obtaining external fetal monitoring may be more difficult. The ability to adequately assess the FHR using external fetal monitors has several factors, including fetal position and maternal body habitus.

Box 2.1: Leopold Maneuvers

First maneuver: Identify the fetal part in the uterine fundus.

- Standing at the patient's side, use the palmar surface of the hand with fingers together to palpate the uterine fundus.
- The fetal head will feel hard, round, and movable, indicating breech presentation.
- The fetal buttocks will feel firm but immovable, indicating vertex presentation.

Second maneuver: Determine the location of the fetal back.

- Use the palmar surface of both hands with one on each side of the maternal abdomen.
- In a step-like fashion, keep one hand firmly in place, using the other hand to palpate from the fundus toward the symphysis pubis. Repeat on the opposite side.
- The fetal back will feel firm and smooth while fetal extremities will feel irregular.

Third maneuver (Pallach grip): Identify the presenting part.

- Using the thumb and fingers of the dominant hand, grasp the presenting part in the lower uterine segment, at the level of the symphysis pubis. Use the other hand at the fundus to stabilize and confirm findings.
- If the presenting part moves upward, the fetus is not engaged in the maternal pelvis.
- This should confirm findings from the first maneuver.

Fourth maneuver: Determine the level of descent of the presenting part.

- Fetal attitude is determined by facing the patient's feet and using both hands on either side of the maternal abdomen.
- Moving the hands toward the pelvic brim, only a small portion of the fetal head will be palpable if fully engaged.
  - If the cephalic prominence or brow is noted on the same side as the fetal extremities, the head is flexed.
  - If the cephalic prominence or brow is noted on the same side as the fetal back, the head is extended.

AUSCULTATION

Auscultation is a method of periodically listening to the fetal heartbeat. Auscultation is done with either a fetoscope or a handheld Doppler device. IA is the technique of listening to and counting the FHR for short periods during labor as opposed to using continuous EFM. Professional organizations, including ACOG and the American College of Nurse-Midwifery (ACNM), recommend that IA be used only to monitor low-risk, uncomplicated pregnancies during labor. "Low risk" has yet to be consistently defined; however, this term generally encompasses patients without meconium staining, intrapartum bleeding, or abnormal or undetermined fetal test results before giving birth or at initial admission. Low risk can also describe patients without increased risk of developing fetal acidemia during labor due to congenital anomalies or fetal growth restriction, as well as patients without maternal conditions that may affect fetal well-being (e.g., prior Cesarean scar, diabetes, and hypertensive disease). No consensus exists regarding the use of oxytocin with IA. Although the evidence suggests that IA is the best way to monitor healthy patients with healthy pregnancies at low risk of complications, many obstetric providers prefer continuous EFM for all patients (Mullins et al., 2017).

Table 2.2 outlines and compares the various auscultation modalities available.

Interpretation of Intermittent Auscultation Findings

Interpretation using IA (Box 2.2) has been adapted from the National Institute of Child Health and Human Development (NICHD)/ACOG three-tier system to reflect the FHR characteristics that may be obtained via IA. The system has been narrowed down to two categories for the purpose of IA. Category I FHR characteristics are normal and reflect adequate fetal oxygenation, predictive of fetal well-being. Category II includes all FHR characteristics that are not normal or not category I. Continuous EFM may be initiated to verify or provide clarity for an indeterminate or abnormal FHR based on IA.

Table 2.2 Fetal Heart Rate Auscultation Modalities Versus EFM

FHR Characteristic	Fetoscope	Handheld Doppler	Continuous EFM
Variability	No	No	Yes
Baseline FHR	Yes	Yes	Yes
Accelerations	Detects increases but cannot quantify as acceleration	Detects increases but cannot quantify as acceleration	Yes
Decelerations	Detects decreases but does not differentiate type of deceleration	Detects decreases but does not differentiate type of deceleration	Yes; differentiates types of decelerations
Rhythm	Yes	Yes	Yes
Double or half counting	May help clarify	No; may double or half count	No; may double or half count
Differentiation between maternal and FHR	Yes	No; may detect maternal HR	No; may detect and record maternal HR

EFM, electronic fetal monitoring; FHR, fetal heart rate.

Source: Modified from ACNM. (2015). Intermittent auscultation for intrapartum fetal heart rate surveillance. *Journal of Midwifery & Women's Health, 60,* 627.

Box 2.2: Interpretation of Intermittent Auscultation

Category I FHR characteristics by IA include all of the following:

■ Normal FHR baseline
■ Regular rhythm
■ Presence of FHR accelerations
■ Absence of FHR decelerations

Category II FHR characteristics by IA include any of the following:

■ Irregular rhythm
■ Presence of FHR decelerations
■ FHR tachycardia
■ FHR bradycardia

FHR, fetal heart rate; IA, intermittent auscultation.

Source: Lyndon, A., & Ali, L. U. (2009). *AWHONN fetal heart rate monitoring: Principles and practices* (4th ed.). Kendall Hunt Publishing.

Recommendations for Auscultation in Labor

To date, there is no consensus nor any studies to determine the optimal frequency of IA during labor. Current recommendations are based on ACNM guidelines and referenced by ACOG (2019). Based on the absence of evidence-based parameters for optimal interval auscultation, current recommendations include auscultation every 15 to 30 minutes during the active phase, every 15 minutes during the second stage prior to the initiation of pushing, and every 5 minutes after the pushing initiation as long as the FHR is normal and no other labor characteristics suggest the need for more frequent monitoring (ACNM, 2015; ACOG, 2010).

Clinical Pearl

While IA is labor intensive, providing the best, evidence-based care to all patients should guide clinical practice over convenience and fear of litigation. It is often underused due to need for increased staffing.

DOPPLER ULTRASOUND

External continuous fetal monitoring is the most common method of assessing fetuses in the United States during labor (Martin et al., 2003), and it often requires the patient to be immobile to obtain accurate readings. In recent years, a portable version of continuous fetal monitoring has been introduced to the market; however, it is not widely used for a variety of reasons. The external fetal monitor detects FHR through the transmission of sound waves and Doppler shifts. Electronic fetal monitors convert the reflected sound waves into electronic signals representing the FHR. This signal is converted via computer processing into an FHR tracing. External monitors are used when the membranes are intact and cannot or should not be ruptured. They are also used in situations when puncture of fetal skin is contraindicated due to concern for vertical transmission of infection, such as in patients with HIV, hepatitis, or herpes simplex. External monitors are also used when the tracing is adequate and minimally invasive techniques are desired. The ultrasound component is attached to the maternal abdomen via a belt at a location where fetal cardiac signals are at their optimum for pickup. EFM is associated with high false-positive rates and inconsistent FHR tracing interpretations, both of which contribute to an inability to accurately predict fetal hypoxia (Alfirevic et al., 2006; Tekin et al., 2008).

FETAL SPIRAL ELECTRODE

Pioneered in the late 1960s, the fetal spiral electrode (FSE) is a form of internal fetal monitoring used during the labor and delivery process that is typically necessary only when external fetal monitoring proves inadequate or to confirm a nonreassuring fetal tracing. For many patients, monitoring the FHR with an external device is sufficient; however, in some cases, the FSE can be an invaluable tool. Guided by a catheter and connected to a spiral wire, the electrode attaches to the fetal scalp to allow for a more precise heart rate reading. Due to the invasive nature of the FSE, this method is often considered a last resort to obtain critical data regarding the well-being of the fetus. The use of an FSE may be indicated when external monitoring cannot provide an adequate continuous tracing of an FHR, such as when:

■ Maternal obesity is a factor.
■ Maternal position must be changed frequently and rapidly.
■ There is a need to distinguish the fetal tracing from the maternal heartbeat.
■ Fetal decelerations are present.

In these situations, an FSE can effectively evaluate fetal heartbeat and its variations—even during uterine contractions—and provide labor and delivery staff with reliable insight into the fetal condition. FSEs detect actual beat-to-beat electrical signals of the fetal heart, whereas external monitoring uses an averaging algorithm, or autocorrelation, to smooth signals generated from the Doppler.

That being said, there are a handful of reasons to avoid using FSEs, and they certainly should not be used routinely. Because an FSE punctures the skin of the fetus, there is a possibility of spreading bloodborne diseases. Therefore, this clinical accessory should be avoided in the presence of maternal HIV, herpes, hepatitis, or other bloodborne diseases that can be transmitted from patient to fetus. Bleeding can also occur at the site of placement, impeding the use of the FSE for fetal monitoring when there is a known or suspected neonatal clotting disorder. Suspected vasa or placenta previa is also a contraindication.

As shown in a 2016 study, the use of an FSE may be associated with a small increased risk of fetal scalp injury, cephalohematoma, and neonatal sepsis. However, these rates were similar to or less than the rates seen with operative vaginal deliveries, with 1.2% of babies receiving a scalp ulcer. The authors of the study concluded that the increased risk of sepsis seen in the study was likely due to the higher-risk nature of patients receiving an FSE (Kawakita et al., 2016). More serious risks to the fetus have been reported, including eyelid laceration, abscess, and even osteomyelitis. However, many of the aforementioned risks and complications can be avoided or minimized by judicious and appropriate use of the FSE for fetal monitoring, proper training, and good technique during placement. Before placing the FSE, ensure that:

■ The membranes are already ruptured.
■ The fetal part is identified and engaged.
■ The patient is at least 2 cm dilated.
■ The placement will avoid the fetal face or genitals.

▶ ANTEPARTUM FETAL SURVEILLANCE METHODS

Antepartum fetal surveillance techniques based on assessment of FHR patterns have been in clinical use for over 6 decades and are used along with real-time ultrasonography and umbilical artery (UA) Doppler studies to evaluate fetal well-being. Antepartum fetal surveillance techniques are routinely used to assess the risk of fetal death in pregnancies complicated by preexisting maternal conditions as well as those in which complications have developed. Several antepartum fetal surveillance techniques are in clinical use, including the nonstress test (NST), contraction stress test (CST), maternal perception of fetal movement, biophysical profile (BPP), modified BPP, and UA Doppler studies.

NONSTRESS TEST

An NST involves the use of external EFM equipment for the purposes of fetal evaluation based on the premise that the fetus is not acidotic or neurologically depressed at a moment in time. FHR reactivity is believed to be a good indicator of normal fetal autonomic function. Loss of reactivity is most commonly associated with a fetal sleep cycle but may result from any cause of central nervous system depression, including fetal acidemia. NSTs are noninvasive, are relatively easy to perform, and may be performed in an office setting to be more cost-efficient. The patient may be positioned in either the semi-Fowler position or the lateral recumbent position. In one small randomized study, it took less time to obtain a reactive NST when patients were placed in the semi-Fowler position (Nathan et al., 2000). The FHR is monitored with an external ultrasound transducer.

NST results are categorized as reactive or nonreactive. The most common definition of a reactive NST is if there are two or more FHR accelerations (as previously defined based on gestational age) within a 20-minute period. The NST should be conducted for at least 20 minutes, but it may be necessary to monitor the tracing for up to 40 minutes to allow for the variations of the fetal sleep-wake cycle. A nonreactive NST is one that lacks sufficient FHR accelerations over a 40-minute period. The NST of the normal preterm fetus is frequently nonreactive: From 24 weeks' to 28 weeks' gestation, up to 50% of NSTs may nonreactive (Bishop, 1981), and from 28 weeks' to 32 weeks' gestation, 15% of NSTs are nonreactive (Druzin et al., 1985; Lavin et al., 1984). The predictive value of NSTs based on a lower threshold for accelerations based on gestational age (10 × 10 as opposed to 15 × 15) has been evaluated in pregnancies at less than 32 weeks' gestation and has been found to sufficiently predict fetal well-being (Cousins et al., 2012; Glantz & Bertoia, 2011). Variable decelerations may be observed in up to half of all NSTs performed (Meis et al., 1986). Variable decelerations that are nonrepetitive and brief (less than 30 seconds) are not associated with fetal compromise or the need for intervention. Repetitive variable decelerations (at least three in 20 minutes), even if mild, have been associated with an increased risk of Cesarean delivery for a nonreassuring intrapartum FHR pattern (Divon et al., 1986; O'Leary et al., 1980). FHR decelerations during an NST that persist for 1 minute or longer are associated with a markedly increased risk of both Cesarean delivery for a nonreassuring fetal status and fetal demise (Bourgeois et al., 1984; Druzin et al., 1981; Pazos et al., 1982). In this setting, the decision to deliver should be made with consideration of whether the benefits outweigh the potential risks of expectant management.

CONTRACTION STRESS TEST

The CST is based on the response of the FHR to uterine contractions. Although it is not routinely used in clinical practice today, clinicians should be educated regarding the procedure, interpretation, and implications of a CST. It is theorized that fetal oxygenation will be transiently worse during a uterine contraction. In the fetus with suboptimal oxygenation, the resulting intermittent worsening in oxygenation will, in turn, lead to the FHR pattern of late decelerations. Uterine contractions may also provoke or highlight a pattern of variable decelerations caused by fetal umbilical cord compression, which may be associated with oligohydramnios.

With the patient in the lateral recumbent position, the FHR and uterine contractions are simultaneously recorded with an external fetal monitor. An adequate uterine contraction pattern is present when at least three contractions persist for at least 40 seconds each in a 10-minute period. Uterine stimulation is not necessary if the patient is having spontaneous uterine contractions of adequate frequency. If fewer than three contractions of 40 seconds' duration occur in 10 minutes, contractions are induced with either nipple stimulation or IV oxytocin (Pitocin). A spontaneous CST can be considered if the adequate number and strength of contractions are noted in the 10-minute time frame. Nipple stimulation is usually successful in inducing an adequate contraction pattern and allows completion of testing in approximately half the time required when IV oxytocin (Pitocin) is used (Huddleston et al., 1984).

The CST is interpreted according to the presence or absence of late FHR decelerations (Freeman et al., 1982). The results of the CST are categorized as follows (ACOG, 2021):

■ Negative—No late or significant variable decelerations
■ Positive—Late decelerations following 50% or more of contractions (even if the contraction frequency is fewer than three in 10 minutes)
■ Equivocal-suspicious—Intermittent late decelerations or significant variable decelerations
■ Equivocal-tachysystole—FHR decelerations that occur in the presence of contractions that are more frequent than every 2 minutes or last longer than 90 seconds
■ Unsatisfactory—Fewer than three contractions in 10 minutes or a tracing that is not interpretable

Relative contraindications to the CST usually include conditions that are associated with an increased risk of preterm labor and delivery, uterine rupture, uterine bleeding, or other conditions in which labor or vaginal delivery are contraindicated. The CST is a safe and effective method of investigating FHR nonreactivity in preterm gestations (Thompson et al., 1990).

FETAL MOVEMENT AND STIMULATION

Fetal movement assessment occurs when the pregnant patient perceives a decrease in fetal movement. The patient counts fetal kicks/movements as a means of antepartum fetal surveillance. A decrease in the maternal perception of fetal movement may precede fetal death, in some cases by several days (Pearson & Weaver, 1976). The optimal number of movements and the ideal duration for counting movements have not been determined; however, numerous protocols have been reported and appear to be acceptable. Perception of 10 distinct movements in a period of up to 2 hours is often considered reassuring. In another approach, patients were instructed to count fetal movements for 1 hour three times per week (Neldam, 1980). The count was considered reassuring if it equaled or exceeded the patient's previously established baseline count. Regardless of the fetal movement approach used, in the absence of a reassuring count, further fetal assessment is recommended.

If fetal stimulation is indicated, vibroacoustic stimulation may elicit FHR accelerations that are valid in the prediction of fetal well-being. Such stimulation offers the advantage of safely reducing the frequency of nonreactive NSTs by 40% and the overall testing time by almost 7 minutes without compromising detection of the acidotic fetus (Clark et al., 1989; Miller et al., 1996; Smith et al., 1986; Tan et al., 2013). To perform vibroacoustic stimulation, the baseline FHR must first be established. The device is then positioned on the maternal abdomen, typically over the fetal head, and a stimulus is applied for 1 to 2 seconds. If vibroacoustic stimulation fails to elicit a response, it may be repeated up to three times for progressively longer durations of up to 3 seconds.

BIOPHYSICAL PROFILE

The BPP consists of an NST combined with four observations made by real-time ultrasonography. It is often used as part of routine antepartum fetal surveillance, as described in Table 2.1, to evaluate a nonreactive NST, or to evaluate patient complaints of decreased fetal movement. Thus, the BPP comprises five components:

1. NST—May be omitted without compromising test validity if the results of all four ultrasound components of the BPP are normal
2. Fetal breathing movements—One or more episodes of rhythmic fetal breathing movements of 30 seconds or more within 30 minutes
3. Fetal movement—Three or more discrete body or limb movements within 30 minutes
4. Fetal tone—One or more episodes of extension of a fetal extremity with return to flexion, or opening or closing of a hand
5. Determination of the amniotic fluid volume—A single deepest vertical pocket greater than 2 cm is considered evidence of adequate amniotic fluid

Each of the five components is assigned a score of either 2 (present) or 0 (not present). A composite score of 8 or 10 is reassuring, a score of 6 is considered equivocal, and a score of 4 or less is abnormal with potential for chronic fetal asphyxia. BPPs with a score of 6 or less require further evaluation and evaluation for delivery. Recommendations should be made based on the overall patient risks and risk-benefit analysis related to potential neonatal outcomes. Regardless of the composite score, oligohydramnios should prompt further evaluation.

MODIFIED BIOPHYSICAL PROFILE

In the late second-trimester or third-trimester fetus, amniotic fluid volume reflects fetal urine production. Placental dysfunction may result in diminished fetal renal perfusion, leading to oligohydramnios (Seeds, 1981). Amniotic fluid volume assessment can therefore be used to evaluate uteroplacental function. This observation fostered the development of what has come to be termed the *modified BPP* as a primary mode of antepartum fetal surveillance. The modified BPP combines the NST, as a short-term indicator of fetal acid-base status, with an amniotic fluid volume assessment, as an indicator of long-term placental function (Clark et al., 1989). Results of the modified BPP are considered normal if the NST is reactive and the amniotic fluid volume is greater than 2 cm in the deepest vertical pocket, and they are considered abnormal if either the NST is nonreactive or the amniotic fluid volume in the deepest vertical pocket is 2 cm or less.

UMBILICAL ARTERY DOPPLER

Doppler ultrasonography is a noninvasive technique used to assess the hemodynamic components of vascular resistance in pregnancies complicated by fetal growth restriction. UA Doppler velocimetry has been adapted for use as a technique of surveillance for a fetus with growth restriction, based on the observation that flow velocity waveforms in the UA of normally growing fetuses differ from those of growth-restricted fetuses. Specifically, the umbilical flow velocity waveform of normally growing fetuses is characterized by high-velocity diastolic flow, whereas in growth-restricted fetuses, there is decreased UA diastolic flow (Erskine & Ritchie, 1985; Gudmundsson & Marsal, 1988; Reuwer et al., 1984). In some cases of severe fetal growth restriction, diastolic flow is absent or even reversed. The perinatal mortality rate in pregnancies with absent end-diastolic flow or reverse end-diastolic flow is significantly increased (Karsdorp et al., 1994). Commonly measured flow indices, based on the characteristics of peak systolic velocity and frequency shift (S), end-diastolic frequency shift (D), and mean peak frequency shift over the cardiac cycle (A), include the following:

- Systolic to diastolic ratio (S/D)
- Resistance index (S–D/S)
- Pulsatility index (S–D/A)

Randomized studies on the utility of UA Doppler velocimetry generally have defined abnormal flow as either absent or reversed end-diastolic flow (REDV; Acharya et al., 2005; Almström et al., 1992; Johnstone et al., 1993). Currently, there is no evidence that UA Doppler velocimetry provides information about fetal well-being in the fetus with normal growth.

▶ TECHNIQUES FOR ASSESSMENT OF UTERINE ACTIVITY

Evaluating uterine activity is a critical part of the clinician's role during the labor process. Multiple assessment techniques are available to clinicians. Despite available technologies, clinicians should remember the value of basic physical assessment.

PALPATION

Another important aspect of the abdominal assessment is palpation of uterine activity. As the uterus contracts, it becomes firmer and denser. This may be assessed using the clinician's fingertips. Aside from uterine activity, abdominal palpation may also be used to assess for uterine tenderness, estimated fetal weight, and fetal movement (Wisner & Holschuh, 2018). Proper palpation should be performed through the entire contraction as well as between contractions to evaluate resting tone. Tips for performing accurate palpation include:

- Assess for the maternal perception of contractions.
- Provide a complete explanation to the patient of why an assessment is being completed, including requesting permission to touch the patient.
- Use the fingertips for palpation, as they are the most sensitive part of the hand.
- Begin palpation near the fundus, as this is typically where contractions are best assessed.
- Firmly but gently attempt to indent the uterus to assess uterine contraction strength.
- Assess contraction frequency by palpating from the beginning of one contraction to the beginning of the next contraction.
- Assess contraction duration by palpating from the onset of uterine firmness until its resolution.
- Assess contraction intensity as mild, moderate, or strong based on the clinician's ability to indent the uterus (Table 2.3).

Table 2.3 Palpation of Uterine Activity

Mild	Moderate	Strong
Easily indented	May be slightly indented	Does not indent
Feels like tip of nose	Feels like a chin	Feels like a forehead

- Assess resting tone as either soft or firm.
- Assess uterine relaxation time, which is the time from the end of one contraction to the start of the next contraction (Lyndon & Wisner, 2021).

Clinical Pearl

Never underestimate the value of palpation and clinician evaluation, despite all of the available technologies.

TOCODYNAMOMETER TRANSDUCER

External tocodynamometers are pressure-sensitive devices used to measure tension across the abdominal wall and detect only approximate contraction frequency and duration. The appearance of contractions by external monitoring may be affected not only by contraction strength but also by maternal habitus, position, gestational age, and monitor location on the abdomen. Placement should be over the area of strongest contraction to measure duration and frequency of uterine contractions. Placement should be determined by clinician palpation and is ideally done over a smooth part of the uterus.

Effective contraction monitoring is often dependent on maternal body habitus. On a patient with a gravid abdomen who is not obese, contractions are often easy to trace and appear very strong. In a patient with excess adipose tissue and obesity, abdominal tightening may be difficult to assess and appear very weak. As a result, it is imperative to use all available assessment methods, including clinician palpation and maternal perception, to guide care during labor while using external monitors.

INTRAUTERINE PRESSURE CATHETER

An IUPC is a sterile device placed through the cervix into the uterus during labor to measure the duration, frequency, and strength of uterine contractions. An IUPC is placed when quantification of contraction strength is desired, typically to assess the adequacy of spontaneous contractions in cases of arrested cervical dilation or to facilitate titration of the oxytocin (Pitocin) dosage during induction or augmentation of labor. Placement of an IUPC can reduce the use of oxytocin (Pitocin) during high-risk labor with signs of fetal distress. An IUPC can provide a more accurate assessment of contraction duration, length, and strength in patients for whom external tocodynamometry does not pick up contractions well, such as in patients with obesity. In cases of FHR decelerations, an IUPC can be used to clarify the relationship between the timing of the deceleration and the contraction. Finally, IUPC placement also allows an amnioinfusion to be performed in cases of severe variable FHR decelerations. An intact fetal membrane is a contraindication to IUPC placement, as the desired location is within the amniotic space. Amniotomy just prior to IUPC placement is acceptable in the absence of contraindications to amniotomy. Maternal infection with communicable diseases, such as HIV or hepatitis B, is also considered a contraindication to internal monitors.

After connection to the appropriate cable, contractions are measured in mmHg and displayed on the monitor in a graphic fashion. With an IUPC in place, Montevideo units (MVUs) can be calculated to assess for adequacy of labor in cases of suspected labor dystocia or during labor induction. MVUs are calculated by subtracting the baseline uterine pressure from the peak uterine pressure of each contraction in a 10-minute window of time and then taking the sum of these pressures. Two hundred MVUs or more is considered adequate for normal labor progression. Routine use of IUPCs is not recommended. A large randomized trial of internal versus external tocodynamometry for monitoring labor showed no difference in rates of operative delivery or fetal outcomes between the two groups. Internal tocodynamometry is more expensive and invasive and should be reserved for specific circumstances (ACOG, 2003).

▶ POTENTIAL MONITORING COMPLICATIONS AND TROUBLESHOOTING

SIGNAL AMBIGUITY

Confusing the maternal heart rate and the FHR when using external EFM is common. When the mix-up is noted and corrected expeditiously, it is unlikely to result in an adverse outcome. Signal ambiguity may arise from faulty Doppler equipment or the inability of the EFM machine to differentiate between maternal heart rate and FHR. It commonly occurs after repositioning the patient, after fetal movement, or during pushing in the second stage when the maternal heart rate may increase to a baseline that is similar to that of the fetus. Signal ambiguity should be suspected when the FHR runs in the low-normal range or when FHR accelerations are noted with greater than 50% of contractions (especially when pushing). Signal ambiguity also should be ruled out when there is an apparent FHR deceleration to the maternal range that does not recover.

Most commonly, recording of the maternal heart rate occurs during the second stage of labor. Early in labor, the normal FHR typically exceeds the basal maternal heart rate. However, in the presence of chorioamnionitis and maternal fever or with the stress of maternal pushing, the maternal heart rate frequently approaches or exceeds that of the FHR. The maximum maternal heart rate can be estimated as 220 bpm minus the maternal age. Thus, the heart rate in a 20-year-old patient may reach rates of 160 to 180 bpm, equivalent to 80% to 90% of the patient's maximum heart rate during second-stage pushing. The external Doppler ultrasound fetal monitor, having a somewhat narrow acoustic window, may lose the focus on the fetal heart as a result of the descent of the fetus, the abdominal shape-altering effect of uterine contractions, and the patient's pushing. During the second stage, EFM may record the maternal heart rate from the uterine arteries. Although some clinicians claim to differentiate the maternal heart rate from the FHR by the "whooshing" maternal uterine artery signal as compared with the "thumping" FHR signal, this auditory assessment is unproven and likely unreliable. In order to differentiate the two, it is important that the initial intervention for an abnormally low FHR is to assess the maternal heart rate and the FHR simultaneously.

Evaluating for suspected signal ambiguity involves two key steps: (1) documentation and verification of the maternal heart rate and (2) definitive documentation of the true FHR. To document the maternal heart rate, manually count the radial pulse for 1 minute or use a pulse oximeter for continuous monitoring. Using a pulse oximeter is a less labor-intensive approach and has the advantage of allowing continuous assessment of the maternal heart rate for comparison. Recording the maternal pulse continuously on the same screen as the FHR enables ongoing differentiation of the patient and fetus in difficult cases, particularly if internal fetal monitoring is not an option (e.g., because of maternal infectious disease, low suspicion for an abnormal FHR pattern, or strong maternal preference against internal monitoring).

POOR FETAL TRACING

The ability to accurately interpret a continuous FHR tracing depends on the quality of data recorded. Unfortunately, the absence of data makes interpretation impossible. This includes both FHR and uterine activity data, since both pieces of information are required for appropriate interpretation of a continuous FHR tracing. Prolonged periods of uninterpretable FHR and uterine activity tracings imply that no one has been attending the patient. If it is difficult to obtain an interpretable FHR tracing, it should be documented in the medical record that ongoing efforts were made to maintain an adequate tracing, including the amount of time spent holding the external monitor, the use of ultrasonography to document the FHR, and plans for potential internal monitoring if not contraindicated.

MONITORING MULTIPLES

The increase in the incidence of multifetal gestations over the last 20 years has intensified the clinical challenge to electronically monitor multiple fetuses. Approximately 5% of pregnancies among patients age 35 to 44 years, and more than 20% of pregnancies in patients age 45 years and older (many due to the use of assisted reproductive technologies), result in multiple gestations (American Society for Reproductive Medicine, 2021). EFM attempts to discriminate between multiple FHRs. Ultrasound may be used to locate each fetus and maximize the likelihood of securing independent tracings. The designation of "Twin A" is usually for the fetus in the lowest portion of the pelvis. Dual-channel electronic fetal monitors allow simultaneous heart rate recordings, which display each FHR in a different color and/or one FHR in a bold line and the other in a faint line. Some electronic monitors use discrimination technology that uses printing of signal marks on the tracing, separate monitoring scales, or artificial separation of single-scale tracings into two separate tracings. Each FHR should be clearly labeled to correlate with the monitoring method and allow differentiation between or among fetuses to avoid the phenomenon of fetal synchronicity associated with monitoring multiples. Documentation should include a description of each FHR tracing. There is no standard requiring separate EFM monitors to evaluate each fetus.

ARTIFACT

Artifact describes irregular variations or the absence of the FHR on a tracing resulting from mechanical limitations of the monitor, electrical interference, or a weak signal appearing on the tracing as gaps or dots (Parer et al., 2018). While all fetal monitors contain a logic system designed to reject artifact, it is still a common clinical occurrence and may result from maternal or fetal movement, in association with clinical intervention, from transducer displacement, or electively as a result of the clinical decision to allow undisturbed maternal rest. When an external Doppler ultrasound transducer is used, gaps or dots may appear when the fetal cardiac signal either is too weak to be continually traced or is not detected. The most common artifact in this scenario is increased variability. When an FSE is used, artifact may appear as irregular lines with various lengths, unlike the regular lines seen with fetal arrhythmias. Other examples of artifact include:

- Half-counting the FHR when it is rapid (over 240 bpm), such as with fetal supraventricular tachycardia (SVT)
- Double-counting during periods of fetal bradycardia
- Recording the maternal heart rate

Troubleshooting should include repositioning the ultrasound transducer, ensuring that an adequate amount of ultrasound gel is used, and checking for proper FSE placement. Occasionally, in medical-legal situations, the presence of what appears to be absent FHR tracing or artifact is alleged to represent the absence of clinician attention to monitoring of the FHR. In fact, this is often a clinical inevitability of external antepartum and intrapartum FHR monitoring that does not necessarily represent clinical disregard nor ability to audibly appreciate the FHR. The question often arises: How much artifact is acceptable to meet the standard of care? To make this decision, providers rely on an evidence-based approach, which incorporates the demands and circumstances of the individual clinical situation, clinical expertise, individualized needs of the patient, and current recommendations for best practice. Management may also be based on recent fetal surveillance, audible findings, maternal-fetal risk status, stage of labor, gestational age, and/or medication use.

FETAL ARRHYTHMIAS

Fetal cardiac ectopy often shows as brief spikes on the fetal monitoring strips during labor. Premature atrial contractions (PACs) appear as upward strokes, while downward strokes represent the compensatory pause. The baseline FHR can be intermittently seen between these upward and downward strokes. If the fetus is experiencing frequent PACs, obtaining an adequate tracing may be difficult. PACs typically have little to no clinical significance and are not considered a sign of fetal hypoxia (Freeman et al., 2012). Fetal premature ventricular contractions (PVCs) are rare, with PACs being 10 times more common (Bravo-Valenzuela et al., 2018). PVCs will also show a vertical spike on the tracing, making them virtually indistinguishable from PACs. Most fetal PVCs are benign and resolve spontaneously. Fetal arrhythmias are differentiated from artifact based on the shape and regularity of spikes. EFM cannot reliably distinguish an atrial arrhythmia from a ventricular arrhythmia (Miller et al., 2017). Differentiation can only be made via fetal echocardiogram, neonatal EKG, and/or neonatal echocardiogram.

CORRECTIVE ACTIONS FOR VARIOUS EXTERNAL EFM PROBLEMS
Erratic Recordings or Gaps on the Tracing Paper

Potential causes for erratic recordings or gaps on the tracing paper include:

- Inadequate conduction of ultrasound signal
- Displaced ultrasound transducer
- Fetal movement or maternal position changes
- Fetal arrhythmias
- Paper not loaded correctly
- Equipment malfunction

Potential corrective actions for erratic recordings or gaps on the tracing paper include:

- Assess for sufficient ultrasound gel on the transducer, applying until a light seal is formed.
- Encourage maternal position changes.
- Check to ensure the belt is snug against the maternal abdomen.
- Reposition the ultrasound transducer over the fetal back, using Leopold maneuvers as needed.
- Distinguish maternal heart rate from FHR by palpation of the maternal radial pulse or applying a pulse oximeter.
- Check all cables and equipment connections, and replace cables as needed.
- Ensure the paper is loaded correctly.
- Apply FSE if clinically indicated and no contraindications are present (Lyndon & Wisner, 2021).

CORRECTIVE ACTIONS FOR VARIOUS FSE PROBLEMS
Intermittent Markings on the FHR Tracing

Potential causes for intermittent markings on the FHR tracing include:

- Artifact
- Failure to detect electrical activity
- Fetal arrhythmia
- Poor monitor connections

Potential corrective actions for intermittent markings on the FHR tracing include:

- Confirm FHR with fetoscope, Doppler, or external ultrasound device.
- Check monitor cables and circuitry and replace cables as needed.
- Turn off logic so as to not mask arrhythmia (Lyndon & Wisner, 2021).

Illegible FHR Tracing

Potential causes for illegible FHR tracing include:

- Artifact
- Faulty electrical connection
- Poor monitor placement
- Incorrect loading or feeding of monitor paper

Potential corrective actions for illegible FHR tracing include:

- Confirm FHR with fetoscope, Doppler, or external ultrasound device.
- Check monitor cables and circuitry and replace cables as needed (Lyndon & Wisner, 2021).

Abnormal Rate on the Tracing/Screen

Potential causes for an abnormal rate on the tracing/screen include:

- Doubling or halving of actual FHR by monitor
- Actual fetal tachycardia, bradycardia, or deceleration
- Interference from maternal signal (fetal demise, FSE placement on maternal cervix)
- Artifact

Potential corrective actions for abnormal rate on the tracing/screen include:

- Confirm FHR with fetoscope, Doppler, or external ultrasound device.
- Verify maternal pulse by palpation and compare with audible signal and printed rate.
- Replace FSE if indicated (Lyndon & Wisner, 2021).

FHR Pattern Compressed

Potential causes for FHR pattern compression include:

- Paper speed or scaling error

Potential corrective actions for FHR pattern compression include:

- Verify paper speed setting (3 cm/min in the United States).
- Check that the correct paper is being used and is loaded correctly (Lyndon & Wisner, 2021).

CORRECTIVE ACTIONS FOR TOCODYNAMOMETER TRANSDUCER PROBLEMS

Contractions not Recording or Inverted Contractions

Potential corrective actions for contractions not recording or inverted contractions include:

- Manually palpate to ensure presence of contractions.
- Confirm tocodynamometer transducer is applied against the abdomen and connected to the monitor.
- Ensure the placement of the tocodynamometer is firm but not tight.
- Test calibration by pushing firmly on the abdominal transducer button; the monitor should display an increase in tone similar to a contraction.
- Palpate the uterus for the area of strongest contraction and reposition the tocodynamometer appropriately.
- Check to be sure the tocodynamometer is not positioned over the maternal umbilicus (Lyndon & Wisner, 2021).

Incomplete Contraction Recording

Potential causes for incomplete contraction recording include:

- Maternal position
- Maternal pushing efforts
- Maternal vomiting

Potential corrective actions for incomplete contraction recording include:

- Consider IUPC placement if clinically indicated and not contraindicated.
- Re-zero baseline resting tone when the uterus is relaxed.
- Palpate the uterus for the area of strongest contraction and reposition the tocodynamometer appropriately.
- Encourage position changes as needed.
- Note clinical events such as episodes of vomiting or when maternal pushing efforts commence (Lyndon & Wisner, 2021).

▶ NEONATAL UMBILICAL CORD BLOOD ANALYSIS

In 1958, James et al. (1958) recognized that umbilical cord blood gas analysis can give an indication of preceding fetal hypoxic stress. It has since become widely accepted that umbilical cord blood gas analysis can provide important information about the past, present, and possibly future condition of the infant. Umbilical cord blood gas analysis is now recommended in all high-risk deliveries by AOCG (2006) and is routine practice following all deliveries in some facilities. It is therefore of increasing clinical and medical-legal importance that clinicians caring for neonates be familiar with the principles and practice of obtaining and interpreting cord blood gas values. Analysis of paired arterial and venous specimens can give insights into the etiology of neonatal acidosis. In combination with other clinical information, normal paired arterial and venous cord blood gas results can usually provide a robust defense against a suggestion that an infant had an intrapartum hypoxic-ischemic event (Armstrong & Stenson, 2007).

INDICATIONS

ACOG (2006) also favors a selective approach, stating that cord blood testing should be applied in the following situations:

- Cesarean delivery for fetal compromise
- Low 5-minute Apgar score
- Severe fetal growth restriction
- Abnormal FHR tracing
- Maternal thyroid disease
- Intrapartum fever
- Multifetal gestation

The lack of consensus among professional organizations is reflected in obstetric practice around the world; some facilities have a selective policy, while others routinely perform cord blood gas analysis at all births. The pros and cons of routine cord blood gas analyses were discussed by Thorp et al. (1996).

Advantages of routine cord blood gas testing include:

- All "damaged babies" will have a cord blood pH on record (important for medical-legal disputes because a normal cord blood pH usually excludes perinatal asphyxia as the cause of brain injury).
- Staff become more proficient in obtaining cord blood samples.
- Process becomes habitual, so less chance of "forgetting" to perform in emergency situations.
- Result may assist with newborn care, should unforeseen problems develop after birth.
- Clinicians gain insight into interpretation of EFM for safe and effective intervention strategies (i.e., the testing has educative value).

Disadvantages of routine cord blood gas testing include:

- More costly than selective policy
- Requires increased staff resources that might simply not be available in some units
- Occasional finding of reduced cord blood pH in a normally healthy, "vigorous" newborn might pose a potential medical-legal concern because it falsely suggests birth asphyxia

Proponents of routine cord blood gas analysis also argue that it can be used as an audit of the effectiveness of the fetal monitoring and intervention strategies used in the unit to prevent significant metabolic acidosis and associated neonatal morbidity and mortality. The prevalence of metabolic acidosis at an obstetric unit, which can only be determined by performing cord blood testing at all births, is thus a valuable safety audit measure. This potential safety audit function of universal cord blood gas testing is addressed by a study that suggests that adoption of a universal testing policy may result in improved perinatal outcomes (White et al., 2010).

Clinical Pearl

Facility policies should address umbilical cord blood sampling related to both process and procedure, as well as inclusion criteria for mandatory collection.

PROCEDURE

The clinical value of cord blood gas analysis lies in its ability to provide objective evidence of asphyxia at the moment of birth. It has been shown to be more reliable in this regard than routine clinical assessment at birth using the Apgar scoring system. Umbilical cord blood analysis is assumed to give a picture of the acid-base balance of the infant at the moment of birth when the umbilical circulation was arrested by clamping of the cord. However, from the time of cord clamping, the umbilical cord blood will demonstrate progressive change in acid-base status due to ongoing placental metabolism and gas exchange if it remains attached to the placenta. Small changes in umbilical pH occur within 60 seconds of delivery (Ullrich & Ackerman, 1972), and over 60 minutes cord arterial or venous pH can fall by more than .2 pH units (Armstrong & Stenson, 2006; Lynn & Beeby, 2006). Similar changes occur in blood sampled from placental surface vessels, except that they are larger and less predictable. These changes are not observed if the cord is doubly clamped at birth, isolating a segment of cord blood from both the placenta and the environment (Lynn & Beeby, 2006).

When there is considerable delay in sampling, it is essential to know whether the sample was taken from isolated cord blood or whether ongoing placental metabolism may have altered the results, making them uninterpretable. It is also important to recognize that the umbilical cord can become obstructed before birth. Restriction of umbilical blood flow causes a progressive widening of the difference between umbilical arterial and venous blood gas values. Martin et al. (2005) showed that term infants with nuchal cords have larger differences in umbilical venous and arterial pH, pCO_2, and pO_2 than those without evidence of cord compression. In contrast, arterial to venous differences are small where there is impairment of the maternal perfusion of the placenta, such as in cases of abruption (Johnson & Richards, 1997). Belai et al. (1998) showed that in severe cases, where the cord arterial pH is less than 7.0, the magnitude of the difference in pCO_2 between the UA and the vein predicts the risk of the infant developing encephalopathy. As a result, it is imperative to sample both arterial and venous blood, especially if a neonate shows signs of distress at delivery. In the presence of cord obstruction, a normal umbilical cord venous blood gas could conceal severe mixed umbilical arterial acidosis in an infant with a high risk of adverse outcome. If the obstruction to the umbilical vessels was sudden and complete and this persisted until the moment of delivery or until fetal death, then the cord gases sampled at birth would give a snapshot of the fetal acid-base balance prior to the obstruction. Both umbilical arterial and venous gases could then be normal despite severe intrapartum asphyxia (Pomerance, 2000). In cases of intrapartum stillbirth and in infants who require considerable resuscitation at delivery, normal cord venous and arterial pH do not exclude acute intrapartum asphyxia. A blood gas sample taken from the infant soon after birth would be expected to show marked acidosis if there had been cord obstruction (Pomerance, 2000).

The umbilical vein is larger and easier to sample from than the UA, and when only a single sample can be obtained because of sampling difficulties, it is likely to be venous. Even when paired samples are obtained, it cannot always be assumed that one is from an artery and one is from the vein. Because fetal carbon dioxide is removed from the umbilical arterial blood in the placenta, umbilical venous blood should have a slightly higher pH and a lower pCO_2 than umbilical arterial blood.

The collection process uses the following general guidelines:

- Use a 1-mL heparinized syringe with a short, small-gauge needle (such as an ABG syringe).
- Use a double-clamped cord segment following delivery.
- Obtain the arterial sample first, as it is often more difficult to obtain and the umbilical vein may help support the umbilical arteries from collapsing. Given this potential difficulty, it is widely recommended that blood from both artery and vein is sampled and analyzed, so that arterial blood results can be validated as truly arterial.
- Avoid air bubbles.
- Label samples and send for analysis immediately. Samples do not need to be placed on ice, as they can remain stable at room temperature for up to an hour without significant changes in pH (Riley & Johnson, 1993; Scheans, 2011; Wallman, 1997).

INTERPRETATION

The pH of umbilical cord blood is determined by the presence of respiratory and metabolic acids. Carbon dioxide diffuses readily across the placenta. It is important to evaluate both the respiratory and the metabolic components of each sample. Normal umbilical cord blood gas values are noted in

Table 2.4. Variations from normal values are reviewed in Table 2.5. Although it is the most commonly discussed component, pH is not an ideal parameter for estimating the cumulative exposure to hypoxia. In contrast, the combination of low pH at birth with other abnormal clinical patterns becomes very strongly predictive of adverse sequelae. Perlman and Risser (1996) showed that a combination of cord pH <7.0, a requirement for intubation, and a 5-minute Apgar score of ≤5 had an 80% positive predictive value for the development of seizures.

Table 2.4 Normal Umbilical Cord Blood Gas Values in Term Infants

Umbilical Cord Vessel	Normal Mean Value Range	Standard Deviation
pH	7.2 to 7.29	7.02 to 7.43
pO_2 (mmHg)	15.1 to 23.7	2.0 to 37.8
pCO_2 (mmHg)	49.2 to 56.3	21.5 to 78.3
Base deficit (mEq/L)	2.7 to 8.3	2.0 to 16.3
HCO_3 (mEq/L)	22.0 to 24.1	14.8 to 29.2

HCO_3, bicarbonate; pCO_2, partial pressure of carbon dioxide; pO_2, partial pressure of oxygen.

Source: Data from Thorp, J. A. (1999, December). Rushing RS: Umbilical cord blood gas analysis. *Obstetrics and Gynecology Clinics of North America, 26*(4), 695–709.

Table 2.5 Significance of Variation From Normal Values

Acidosis Type	pH	pO_2	pCO_2	HCO_3	Base Deficit
Respiratory	Low	Varies	High	Normal	Normal
Metabolic	Low	Low	Normal	Low	High
Mixed	Low	Low	High	Low	High

HCO_3, bicarbonate; pCO_2, partial pressure of carbon dioxide; pO_2, partial pressure of oxygen.

Source: Data from Gilstrap, L. III, Leveno, K., Burris, J., Williams, M., & Little, B. (1989). Diagnosis of birth asphyxia on the basis of fetal pH, Apgar score, and newborn cerebral dysfunction. *American Journal of Obstetrics and Gynecology, 161*(3), 825–830. https://doi.org/10.1016/0002-9378(89)90410-9; Helwig, J. T., Parer, J. T., Kilpatrick, S. J., & Laros, R. K. Jr. (1996). Umbilical cord blood acid-base state: What is normal? *American Journal of Obstetrics and Gynecology, 174*(6), 1807–1814. https://doi.org/10.1016/s0002-9378(96)70214-4.

When paired cord blood gas samples produce results that are so similar that it is physiologically implausible and statistically unlikely that they came from an artery and a vein, they should be interpreted in the same way as if they were a single vessel sample (Pomerance, 1999), and it is most likely that they came from the umbilical vein. They do not then exclude the possibility of notable umbilical arterial acidosis, particularly if the rest of the clinical picture points toward this. Low cord pH in infants who are vigorous at birth and free of cardiopulmonary compromise does not indicate an increased risk of adverse outcome. Infants with pH <7.0 at birth who are not vigorous are at high risk of adverse outcome. Identification of infants at risk of encephalopathy is especially important now that early intervention is being considered. In this respect, cord pH and base excess alone are poor predictors of outcome (Winkler et al., 1991).

Significant metabolic acidosis, widely defined as cord arterial blood pH <7.0 and base excess ≤12.0 mmol/L (base deficit ≥12.0 mmol/L), occurs in around .5% to 1% of deliveries (van den Berg et al., 1996; Ross & Gala, 2002; White et al., 2010). The severe intrapartum hypoxia that this degree of cord metabolic acidosis reflects is associated with increased risk of hypoxic brain-cell injury and associated hypoxic-ischemic encephalopathy (HIE). HIE is a neurological condition caused by perinatal asphyxia. Symptoms among affected neonates include hypotonia, poor feeding, respiratory difficulties, seizures, and reduced level of consciousness. Eventual outcome depends on severity and site of brain injury. Those with mild HIE survive with usually little or no long-term consequences, but most of those with moderate to severe HIE either die during the neonatal period or survive with severe and permanent neurological and/or psychological deficit, while cerebral palsy is an outcome for others.

FACTORS IMPACTING RESULTS

Infants born by elective Cesarean section without labor have results that are closer to normal adult values (higher pH, pO_2, base excess, and bicarbonate and lower pCO_2), as do infants born of multiparous patients (Daniel et al., 1998; Riley & Johnson, 1993). Regional anesthesia, particularly spinal anesthesia, is associated with increased incidence of cord blood acidosis (Roberts et al., 1995). Sympathetic blockade reduces uteroplacental perfusion. The resultant carbon dioxide retention is manifested by predominantly respiratory acidosis, but there is no evidence that this affects clinical outcome. The presence of a true knot of the cord seldom seems to cause a problem (Maher & Conti, 1996).

Although placental infection is associated with cerebral palsy in both term and preterm infants, the mechanism appears to be largely independent of hypoxia-ischemia (Perlman, 1997; Wu & Colford, 2000). Chorioamnionitis does not appear to influence cord blood pH or base excess (Graham et al., 2004). The pO_2 and pCO_2 values may provide further clues to the interpretation of the clinical picture and help to exclude inaccurate results. The base excess should still provide a reliable measure for metabolic acidosis; however, it may not be possible to determine whether the specimen is arterial or venous. The lower limit of carbon dioxide is less informative because pregnant patients can spontaneously hyperventilate to a low pCO_2 level. In the absence of compromise to the placental perfusion by the pregnant patient and the fetus, there is a linear relationship between maternal and fetal pCO_2 (Cook, 1984). However, the changes in fetal pH associated with brief hyperventilation are small. Maternal hyperventilation lowers fetal pO_2 (Cook, 1984).

▶ KEY POINTS

- Understanding the use and value of various methods of fetal monitoring allows clinicians to use the best resources for each patient situation.
- The goal of antepartum fetal surveillance is to provide useful information related to fetal oxygenation status.
- Successful troubleshooting strategies related to fetal monitoring errors allow clinicians the ability to provide better care for all patients.
- Umbilical cord gas analysis provides clinicians with valuable information related to fetal status. Understanding normal values and the variations related to both respiratory and metabolic disturbances is imperative to understanding neonatal outcomes.

CASE STUDY

Shannon is a 28-year-old G3P0111 patient at 39 weeks and 1 day's gestation presenting to labor and delivery after a nonreactive NST and BPP 6/10. Sterile vaginal examination is 3/80/-2 with intact amniotic membranes. The patient has no underlying medical history. The pregnancy has been complicated by a suspected fetal arrhythmia. The patient has not had a fetal echocardiogram. During the initial EFM tracing, significant artifact is noted.

Answer the following questions, and then see the Case Study Answers for correct answers.

1. What are the options for obtaining an accurate fetal tracing?

2. Following artificial rupture of membranes (AROM) with clear fluid, SVE 5/80/-2 with recurrent variable decelerations is noted. What interventions should the clinician consider to improve the fetal tracing?

(See answers next page.)

CASE STUDY ANSWERS

1. The options for obtaining an accurate fetal tracing are:
   - AROM with placement of FSE
   - Turning off logic on fetal monitor

2. The interventions the clinician should consider are:
   - Priority assessment is to evaluate for umbilical cord prolapse following AROM. If no prolapse is present, move forward with additional interventions. If umbilical cord prolapse is noted, maintain vaginal hand to relieve cord compression and proceed with emergent Cesarean delivery.
   - Maternal position changes.
   - Amnioinfusion.

⬤ KNOWLEDGE CHECK: CHAPTER 2

1. To be considered reactive at 33 weeks' gestation, a nonstress test (NST) must include:
   A) Two 10 × 10 accelerations in a 20-minute period
   B) Two 15 × 15 accelerations in a 20-minute period
   C) Two 15 × 15 accelerations in a 40-minute period

2. A 41-year-old patient at 35 weeks and 4 days' gestation with an otherwise uncomplicated pregnancy presents for routine antepartum testing and has a nonreactive nonstress test (NST). The *next* step should be to:
   A) Admit for delivery
   B) Complete a biophysical profile (BPP)
   C) Repeat the NST in 1 week

3. A modified biophysical profile (BPP) includes a nonstress test (NST) and a/an:
   A) Contraction stress test
   B) Ultrasound assessment of amniotic fluid
   C) Ultrasound assessment of fetal movement

4. The clinician is evaluating a patient after the completion of a biophysical profile (BPP). The clinician suspects chronic fetal asphyxia because the score is less than:
   A) 6
   B) 8
   C) 10

5. Interpreting a contraction stress test (CST) requires a *minimum* of how many contractions in a 10-minute window?
   A) 2
   B) 3
   C) 4

6. Which of the following is *not* an indication for antepartum fetal testing?
   A) Gestational diabetes
   B) History of gestational hypertension
   C) History of stillbirth at 33 weeks

7. A 34-week-old fetus is having a nonstress test (NST). The baseline fetal heart rate (FHR) is 135 beats per minute (bpm). The clinician has decided to use vibroacoustic stimulation to reduce the length of time needed to obtain a reactive tracing. Fetal well-being would be indicated by:
   A) One acceleration to 150 bpm
   B) Two accelerations to 145 bpm
   C) Two accelerations to 150 bpm

8. Cord blood gases from one of the umbilical arteries best represent the status of:
   A) Fetal acid-base balance
   B) Maternal oxygenation
   C) Placental function

9. Which fetal heart rate (FHR) tracing features must be assessed to distinguish arrhythmias from artifact?
   A) Shape and regularity of spikes
   B) Spikes and baseline
   C) Spikes and variability

10. A negative contraction stress test (CST) is one in which:
    A) Late decelerations are noted with <50% of contractions
    B) No contractions are noted
    C) No late decelerations are noted

(See answers next page.)

1. B) Two 15 × 15 accelerations in a 20-minute period

In order to be considered reactive at any gestational age ≥32 weeks or in any patient who has previously had 15 × 15 accelerations prior to 32 weeks' gestation, an NST tracing must have at least 15 × 15 accelerations in a 20-minute period. In a patient <32 weeks who has never had documented 15 × 15 accelerations, 10 × 10 accelerations are considered reactive.

2. B) Complete a biophysical profile (BPP)

Following a nonreactive NST in the absence of other risk factors, the next step should be a BPP for additional evaluation of fetal well-being. Given that an NST is often only 20 minutes, a fetal sleep cycle is possible. A BPP can then guide further management. In the absence of other risk factors, admission for delivery of a preterm infant is not yet indicated without additional testing. A repeat NST in 1 week is indicated; however, it is not the next step. The patient requires additional evaluation at this time.

3. B) Ultrasound assessment of amniotic fluid

A modified BPP includes an NST and ultrasound assessment of the amniotic fluid index. Ultrasound assessment of fetal movement is part of a full BPP. A contraction stress test (CST) is not part of either a modified or a full BPP.

4. A) 6

A BPP score of less than 6 is concerning for fetal asphyxia. Biophysical profile scores of 8 and 10 are both reassuring.

5. B) 3

Interpreting a CST requires at least three contractions in a 10-minute window; fewer than three is inadequate for interpretation.

6. B) History of gestational hypertension

While a history of stillbirth at 33 weeks and gestational diabetes are indications for antepartum fetal testing due to the increased risk of morbidity and mortality, a previous history of gestational hypertension is not an indication for antepartum testing.

7. C) Two accelerations to 150 bpm

Fetal well-being is indicated on an NST when there are at least two accelerations at least 15 bpm above baseline. With a baseline FHR of 135 bpm, FHR increases must be at least 150 bpm to qualify as accelerations at 34 weeks' gestational age.

8. A) Fetal acid-base balance

Cord blood gases obtained from the UA are used for analysis of fetal acid-base balance. Maternal oxygenation is best assessed through the use of pulse oximetry or maternal arterial blood gas. Placental function is not directly measured through umbilical cord blood sampling.

9. A) Shape and regularity of spikes

Fetal arrhythmias are differentiated from artifact based on the shape and regularity of the spikes. Variability and baseline are often very difficult to determine in the presence of a fetal arrhythmia.

10. C) No late decelerations are noted

Criteria for a negative CST include the absence of late decelerations with at least three contractions in a 10-minute period. Presence of any late decelerations indicates a positive CST. Contractions are required to have an adequate CST.

11. How long may a standard nonstress test (NST) be extended in a term-gestation pregnancy if not initially reactive?
    A) From the initial 20 minutes to 40 minutes
    B) From the initial 20 minutes to 60 minutes
    C) From the initial 40 minutes to 60 minutes

12. Which is the most appropriate application of vibroacoustic stimulation during a nonstress test (NST)?
    A) Having the patient place the stimulator anywhere on the abdomen
    B) Placing the stimulator after the fetal heart rate (FHR) baseline is established
    C) Placing the stimulator on the maternal fundus

13. A patient being monitored externally has a suspected fetal arrhythmia. The most appropriate action is to:
    A) Insert a fetal spiral electrode (FSE) and turn off logic
    B) Turn logic on if an external monitor is in place
    C) Use a Doppler to evaluate the ventricular rate

14. The ultrasound transducer on an electronic fetal monitor measures the:
    A) Electrical signal of the fetal heart
    B) Mechanical movements of the fetal heart reflected off sound waves
    C) R-to-R interval of the fetal heart rate tracing

15. The purpose of autocorrelation in external monitoring is to:
    A) Compare incoming waveforms
    B) Decrease signal noise levels
    C) Distinguish fetal from maternal heart rate

16. Palpating the uterus is best performed using the clinician's:
    A) Back of hand
    B) Fingertips
    C) Palmar surface

17. The area of maximum intensity of the fetal heart rate (FHR) is typically the fetal:
    A) Abdomen
    B) Back
    C) Chest

18. Which is the most sensitive method for uterine activity assessment?
    A) Clinician palpation
    B) Intrauterine pressure catheter (IUPC)
    C) Maternal perception

19. Which method of assessing the fetal heart rate (FHR) allows the clinician to hear the opening and closing of the heart valves, which helps detect dysrhythmias?
    A) Fetal spiral electrode (FSE)
    B) Fetoscope
    C) Ultrasound transducer

20. The tocodynamometer is unreliable for assessment of a contraction's:
    A) Duration
    B) Frequency
    C) Intensity

21. When monitoring a patient during labor, the clinician notices an abnormally low fetal heart rate (FHR) on the monitor. The *first* intervention should be to:
    A) Compare maternal pulse simultaneously with FHR
    B) Prepare for an emergent Cesarean delivery
    C) Remove the fetal monitor

(*See answers next page.*)

11. A) From the initial 20 minutes to 40 minutes
A standard NST is 20 minutes; however, it may be extended up to 40 minutes to account for a fetal sleep cycle.

12. B) Placing the stimulator after the fetal heart rate (FHR) baseline is established
Vibroacoustic stimulation is used to elicit fetal movement leading to FHR accelerations. The most appropriate placement is over the fetal head, not necessarily the maternal fundus, and not at the whim of the patient.

13. A) Insert a fetal spiral electrode (FSE) and turn off logic
Inserting an FSE and turning off logic may allow the clinician to differentiate artifact from a fetal arrhythmia. All machines have logic on as a default setting and are not useful without an internal monitor.

14. B) Mechanical movements of the fetal heart reflected off sound waves
The ultrasound transducer on an electronic monitor measures the mechanical movements of the fetal heart reflected off sound waves. Electrical signals of the fetal heart cannot be measured by ultrasound.

15. A) Compare incoming waveforms
The purpose of autocorrelation in external monitoring is to compare incoming waveforms, analyze them, and produce a fetal heart rate (FHR) tracing. While autocorrelation does attempt to decrease artifact, it does not decrease the signal noise level. Maternal and FHRs must be distinguished through clinician assessment.

16. B) Fingertips
The fingertips are the most sensitive part of the human hand; therefore, they are best for clinicians to use to perform palpation.

17. B) Back
The FHR is best heard over the area of maximum intensity, which is typically the fetal back because the fetal back is typically closest to the maternal abdominal wall. Since a fetus is typically curled up, the chest is more difficult to access, as it is farther from the maternal abdominal wall. The fetal heart is not located in the abdomen; therefore, it cannot be the area of maximum intensity.

18. B) Intrauterine pressure catheter (IUPC)
IUPCs are more accurate and precise than both clinician palpation and maternal perception. An IUPC provides objective data, while both clinician palpation and maternal perception provide subjective data.

19. B) Fetoscope
Only a fetoscope allows the clinician to hear the opening and closing of the heart valves.

20. C) Intensity
The tocodynamometer is reliable in the assessment of contraction duration and frequency but not intensity. An intrauterine pressure catheter (IUPC) is needed for the accurate assessment of contraction intensity.

21. A) Compare maternal pulse simultaneously with fetal heart rate (FHR)
If an abnormally low FHR is noted on fetal monitoring, the first step should be to compare the maternal pulse simultaneously with the FHR, which can be done through palpation of the maternal radial pulse or via pulse oximeter.

22. Which of the following situations is appropriate for use of vibroacoustic stimulation?
    A) G1P0 patient at 38 weeks and 1 day's gestation undergoing a nonstress test (NST) without contractions. Fetal heart rate (FHR) baseline 140 beats per minute (bpm), minimal variability for 45 minutes. No accelerations. No decelerations.
    B) G2P1001 patient at 40 weeks and 3 days' gestation undergoing an NST with occasional contractions without cervical change. FHR baseline 150 bpm, moderate variability. Prolonged deceleration to 60 bpm lasting 8 minutes.
    C) G3P1011 patient at 37 weeks and 6 days' gestation with frequent contractions without cervical change. FHR baseline 180 bpm, moderate variability. No accelerations. Late decelerations.

23. Which of the following fetal heart rate (FHR) characteristics can be determined using a handheld Doppler?
    A) Baseline
    B) Variability
    C) Type of decelerations

24. The following arterial umbilical cord gas results are obtained after delivery of a term infant: pH 7.09, partial pressure of carbon dioxide (pCO_2) 70, partial pressure of oxygen (pO_2) 25, bicarbonate (HCO_3) 29, and base excess −10. These results are most consistent with which type of acidosis?
    A) Metabolic
    B) Mixed
    C) Respiratory

25. If the pH is low, what other blood gas parameter is used to determine if acidosis is respiratory versus metabolic?
    A) Bicarbonate (HCO_3)
    B) Partial pressure of carbon dioxide (pCO_2)
    C) Partial pressure of oxygen (pO_2)

(See answers next page.)

22. A) G1P0 patient at 38 weeks and 1 day's gestation undergoing a nonstress test (NST) without contractions. Fetal heart rate (FHR) baseline 140 beats per minute (bpm), minimal variability for 45 minutes. No accelerations. No decelerations.

A patient with minimal variability, no accelerations, and no decelerations is an appropriate candidate for vibroacoustic stimulation. Patients with decelerations are not appropriate candidates for vibroacoustic stimulation because additional evaluation will be required beyond an NST.

23. A) Baseline

Only the baseline FHR and presence or absence of accelerations and decelerations can be determined using a handheld Doppler. FHR variability and type of deceleration cannot be determined using a handheld Doppler.

24. C) Respiratory

In an uncomplicated delivery, normal arterial pH is ≥7.10, with preterm newborns having a higher pH. A pH of 7.09 indicates acidosis. Normal arterial pO_2 is >20, and normal pCO_2 is <60 mmHg. The normal pO_2 and high pCO_2 are consistent with respiratory acidosis. A base excess of >−12 and a base deficit of <12 are considered normal.

25. B) Partial pressure of carbon dioxide (pCO_2)

The pH, base excess, and pCO_2 of arterial blood flowing through the umbilical cord provide valuable objective evidence of the neonatal metabolic condition at the time of delivery. If the pH is low, the pCO_2 may be used to determine if the acidosis is respiratory versus metabolic.

▶ REFERENCES

Acharya, G., Wilsgaard, T., Berntsen, G. K., Maltau, J. M., & Kiserud, T. (2005). Reference ranges for serial measurements of umbilical artery Doppler indices in the second half of pregnancy. *American Journal of Obstetrics and Gynecology, 192*(3), 937–944. https://doi.org/10.1016/j.ajog.2004.09.019

Alfirevic, Z., Devane, D., & Gyte, G. M. (2006). Continuous cardiotocography (CTG) as a form of electronic fetal monitoring (EFM) for fetal assessment during labour. *The Cochrane Database of Systematic Reviews,* (3), CD006066. https://doi.org/10.1002/14651858.CD006066

Almström, H., Axelsson, O., Cnattingius, S., Ekman, G., Maesel, A., Ulmsten, U., Arström, K., & Marsál, K. (1992). Comparison of umbilical-artery velocimetry and cardiotocography for surveillance of small-for-gestational-age fetuses. *Lancet, 340*(8825), 936–940. https://doi.org/10.1016/0140-6736(92)92818-z

American College of Nurse-Midwives. (2015). Intermittent auscultation for intrapartum fetal heart rate surveillance: American College of Nurse-Midwives. *Journal of Midwifery & Women's Health, 60*(5), 626–632. https://doi.org/10.1111/jmwh.12372

American College of Obstetrics and Gynecology. (2003). ACOG practice bulletin 49. Dystocia and augmentation of labor. *Obstetrics and Gynecology, 102*(6), 1445–1454. https://doi.org/10.1016/j.obstetgynecol.2003.10.011

American College of Obstetrics and Gynecology. (2006). ACOG committee opinion 348. Umbilical cord blood gas and acid-base analysis. *Obstetrics and Gynecology, 108*(5), 1319–1322.

American College of Obstetrics and Gynecology. (2009). ACOG practice bulletin 106. Intrapartum fetal heart rate monitoring: Nomenclature, interpretation, and general management principles. *Obstetrics and Gynecology, 114*(1), 192–202. https://doi.org/10.1097/AOG.0b013e3181aef106

American College of Obstetrics and Gynecology. (2010). ACOG practice bulletin 116. Management of intrapartum fetal heart rate tracing. *Obstetrics and Gynecology, 116*(5), 1232–1240. https://doi.org/10.1097/AOG.0b013e3182004fa9

American College of Obstetrics and Gynecology. (2019). ACOG committee opinion 766. Approaches to limit intervention during labor and birth. *Obstetrics and Gynecology, 133*(2), e164–e173. https://doi.org/10.1097/AOG.0000000000003074

American College of Obstetrics and Gynecology. (2021). ACOG practice bulletin 229. Antepartum fetal surveillance. *Obstetrics and Gynecology, 137*(6), e116–e127. https://doi.org/10.1097/AOG.0000000000004410

American Society for Reproductive Medicine. (2021). *Oversight of assisted reproductive technology.* https://www.asrm.org/globalassets/_asrm/advocacy-and-policy/oversiteofart.pdf

Armstrong, L., & Stenson, B. (2006). Effect of delayed sampling on umbilical cord arterial and venous lactate and blood gases in clamped and unclamped vessels. *Achieves of Disease in Childhood Fetal and Neonatal Edition, 91*(5), F430–F434. https://doi.org/10.1136/adc.2005.086744

Armstrong, L., & Stenson, B. (2007). Use of umbilical cord blood gas analysis in the assessment of the newborn. *Achieves of Disease in Childhood Fetal and Neonatal Edition, 92*(6), F430–F434. https://doi.org/10.1136/adc.2006.099846

Belai, Y., Goodwin, T. M., Durand, M., Greenspoon, J. S., Paul, R. H., & Walther, F. J. (1998). Umbilical arteriovenous PO_2 and PCO_2 differences and neonatal morbidity in term infants with severe acidosis. *American Journal of Obstetrics and Gynecology, 178*(1), 13–19. https://doi.org/10.1016/s0002-9378(98)70619-2

Bishop, E. H. (1981). Fetal acceleration test. *American Journal of Obstetrics and Gynecology, 141*(8), 905–909. https://doi.org/10.1016/s0002-9378(16)32682-5

Bourgeois, F. J., Thiagarajah, S., & Harbert, G. M. Jr. (1984). The significance of fetal heart rate decelerations during nonstress testing. *American Journal of Obstetrics and Gynecology, 150*(2), 213–216. https://doi.org/10.1016/s0002-9378(84)80018-6

Bravo-Valenzuela, N., Rocha, L., Machado Nardozza, L., & Araujo Juior, E. (2018). Fetal cardiac arrythmias: Current evidence. *Annals in Pediatric Cardiology, 11*(2), 148–163. https://doi.org/10.4103/apc.APC_134_17

Chen, H. Y., Chauhan, S. P., Ananth, C. V., Vintzileos, A. M., & Abuhamad, A. Z. (2011). Electronic fetal heart rate monitoring and its relationship to neonatal and infant mortality in the United States. *American Journal of Obstetrics & Gynecology, 204,* 491.e1–491.e10. https://doi.org/10.1016/j.ajog.2011.04.024

Clark, S. L., Sabey, P., & Jolley, K. (1989). Nonstress testing with acoustic stimulation and amniotic fluid volume assessment: 5973 tests without unexpected fetal death. *American Journal of Obstetrics and Gynecology, 160*(3), 694–697. https://doi.org/10.1016/s0002-9378(89)80062-6

Cook, P. T. (1984). The influence on fetal outcome of maternal carbon dioxide tension at caesarean section under general anaesthesia. *Anaesthesia and Intensive Care, 12*(4), 296–302. https://doi.org/10.1177/0310057X8401200402

Cousins, L. M., Poeltler, D. M., Faron, S., Catanzarite, V., Daneshmand, S., & Casele, H. (2012). Nonstress testing at ≤32.0 weeks' gestation: A randomized trial comparing different assessment criteria. *American Journal of Obstetrics and Gynecology, 207*(4), 311.e1–311.e3117. https://doi.org/10.1016/j.ajog.2012.06.032

Daniel, Y., Fait, G., Lessing, J. B., Jaffa, A., Gull, I., Shenav, M., Peyser, M. R., & Kupferminc, M. J. (1998). Umbilical cord blood acid-base values in uncomplicated term vaginal breech deliveries. *Acta Obstetricia Et Gynecologica Scandinavica, 77*(2), 182–185.

Divon, M., Brustman, L., Anyaegbunam, A., & Langer, O. (1986). The significance of antepartum variable decelerations. *American Journal of Obstetrics and Gynecology, 155*, 707–710. https://doi.org/10.1016/S0002-9378(86)80003-5

Druzin, M. L., Fox, A., Kogut, E., & Carlson, C. (1985). The relationship of the nonstress test to gestational age. *American Journal of Obstetrics and Gynecology, 153*(4), 386–389. https://doi.org/10.1016/0002-9378(85)90075-4

Druzin, M. L., Gratacós, J., Keegan, K. A., & Paul, R. H. (1981). Antepartum fetal heart rate testing. VII. The significance of fetal bradycardia. *American Journal of Obstetrics and Gynecology, 139*(2), 194–198. https://doi.org/10.1016/0002-9378(81)90445-2

Erskine, R. L. & Ritchie, J. W. (1985). Umbilical artery blood flow characteristics in normal and growth retarded fetuses. *British Journal of Obstetrics and Gynaecology, 92*(6), 605–610. https://doi.org/10.1111/j.1471-0528.1985.tb01399.x

Freeman, R. K., Anderson, G., & Dorchester, W. (1982). A prospective multi-institutional study of antepartum fetal heart rate monitoring. I. Risk of perinatal mortality and morbidity according to antepartum fetal heart rate test results. *American Journal of Obstetrics and Gynecology, 143*(7), 771–777. https://doi.org/10.1016/0002-9378(82)90008-4

Freeman, R. K., Garite, T., Nageotte, M., & Miller, L. (2012). *Fetal heart rate monitoring* (4th ed.). Wolters-Kluwer.

Gilstrap, L. III, Leveno, K., Burris, J., Williams, M., & Little, B. (1989). Diagnosis of birth asphyxia on the basis of fetal pH, Apgar score, and newborn cerebral dysfunction. *American Journal of Obstetrics and Gynecology, 161*(3), 825–830. https://doi.org/10.1016/0002-9378(89)90410-9

Glantz, J. C., & Bertoia, N. (2011). Preterm nonstress testing: 10-beat compared with 15-beat criteria. *Obstetrics and Gynecology, 118*(1), 87–93. https://doi.org/10.1097/AOG.0b013e31821d85e5

Graham, E., Holcroft, C., Rai, K, Donohue, P., & Allen, M. (2004). Neonatal cerebral white matter injury in preterm infants is associated with culture positive infections and only rarely with metabolic acidosis. *American Journal of Obstetrics and Gynecology, 191*(4), 1305–1310. https://doi.org/10.1016/j.ajog.2004.06.058

Gudmundsson, S., & Marsal, K. (1988). Umbilical and uteroplacental blood flow velocity waveforms in pregnancies with fetal growth retardation. *European Journal of Obstetrics, Gynecology, and Reproductive Biology, 27*(3), 187–196. https://doi.org/10.1016/0028-2243(88)90122-0

Helwig, J. T., Parer, J. T., Kilpatrick, S. J., & Laros, R. K. Jr. (1996). Umbilical cord blood acid-base state: What is normal? *American Journal of Obstetrics and Gynecology, 174*(6), 1807–1814. https://doi.org/10.1016/s0002-9378(96)70214-4

Huddleston, J. F., Sutliff, G., & Robinson, D. (1984). Contraction stress test by intermittent nipple stimulation. *Obstetrics and Gynecology, 63*(5), 669–673.

James, L. S., Weisbrot, I. M., Prince, C. E., Holaday, D. A., & Apgar, V. (1958). The acid-base status of human infants in relation to birth asphyxia and the onset of respiration. *The Journal of Pediatrics, 52*(4), 379–394. https://doi.org/10.1016/s0022-3476(58)80058-x

Johnson, J., & Richards, D. (1997). The etiology of fetal acidosis as determined by umbilical cord acid-base studies. *American Journal of Obstetrics and Gynecology, 177*(2), 74–80.

Johnstone, F. D., Prescott, R., Hoskins, P., Greer, I. A., Mcglew, T., & Compton, M. (1993). The effect of introduction of umbilical Doppler recordings to obstetric practice. *British Journal of Obstetrics and Gynaecology, 100*(8), 733–741. https://doi.org/10.1111/j.1471-0528.1993.tb1422.x

Karsdorp, V. H., van Vugt, J. M., van Geijn, H. P., Kostense, P. J., Arduini, D., Montenegro, N., & Todros, T. (1994). Clinical significance of absent or reversed end diastolic velocity waveforms in umbilical artery. *Lancet*, *344*(8938), 1664–1668. https://doi.org/10.1016/s0140 -6736(94)90457-x

Kawakita, T., Reddy, U. M., Landy, H. J., Iqbal, S. N., Huang, C. C., & Grantz, K. L. (2016). Neonatal complications associated with use of fetal scalp electrode: A retrospective study. *BJOG: An International Journal of Obstetrics and Gynaecology*, *123*(11), 1797–1803. https://doi.org/10.1111/ 1471-0528.13817

Lavin, J. P. Jr., Miodovnik, M., & Barden, T. P. (1984). Relationship of nonstress test reactivity and gestational age. *Obstetrics and Gynecology*, *63*(3), 338–344.

Lyndon, A., & Wisner, K. (2021). *AWHONN fetal heart rate monitoring: Principles and practices* (6th ed.). Kendall Hunt Publishing.

Lynn, A., & Beeby, P. (2006). Cord and placenta arterial gas analysis: The accuracy of delayed sampling. *Achieves of Disease in Childhood Fetal and Neonatal Edition*, *92*(4), F281–F285. https://doi.org/10.1136/adc.2006.103358

Maher, J., & Conti, J. (1996). A comparison of umbilical cord blood gas values between newborns with and without true knots. *Obstetrics and Gynecology*, *88*(5), 863–866. https://doi .org/10.1016/0029-7844(96)00313-4

Martin, J. A., Hamilton, B. E., Sutton, P. D., Ventura, S. J., Menacker, F., & Munson, M. L. (2003). Births: Final data for 2002. *National Vital Statistics Reports*, *52*(10), 1–113.

Martin, G. C., Green, R. S., & Holzman, I. R. (2005). Acidosis in newborns with nuchal cords and normal Apgar scores. *Journal of Perinatology*, *25*(3), 162–165. https://doi.org/10.1038 /sj.jp.7211238

Meis, P. J., Ureda, J. R., Swain, M., Kelly, R. T., Penry, M., & Sharp, P. (1986). Variable decelerations during nonstress tests are not a sign of fetal compromise. *American Journal of Obstetrics and Gynecology*, *154*(3), 586–590. https://doi.org/10.1016/0002-9378(86)90606-x

Miller, D. A., Rabello, Y. A., & Paul, R. H. (1996). The modified biophysical profile: Antepartum testing in the 1990s. *American Journal of Obstetrics and Gynecology*, *174*(3), 812–817. https://doi .org/10.1016/s0002-9378(96)70305-8

Miller, L. A., Miller, D. A., & Cypher, R. L. (2017). *Fetal monitoring: A multidisciplinary approach* (8th ed.). Elsevier.

Mullins, E., Lees, C., & Brocklehurst, P. (2017). Is continuous electronic fetal monitoring useful for all women in labour? *BMJ (Clinical Research Ed.)*, *359*, j5423. https://doi.org/10.1136/bmj .j5423

Nathan, E. B., Haberman, S., Burgess, T., & Minkoff, H. (2000). The relationship of maternal position to the results of brief nonstress tests: A randomized clinical trial. *American Journal of Obstetrics & Gynecology*, *182*(5), 1070–1072. https://doi.org/10.167/mob.2000.105443

Neldam, S. (1980). Fetal movements as an indicator of fetal wellbeing. *Lancet*, *1*(8180), 1222–1224. https://doi.org/10.1016/s0140-6736(80)91681-5

O'Leary, J. A., Andrinopoulos, G. C., & Giordano, P. C. (1980). Variable decelerations and the non-stress test: An indication of cord compromise. *American Journal of Obstetrics and Gynecology*, *137*(6), 704–706. https://doi.org/10.1016/s0002-9378(15)33245-2

Parer, J., King, T., & Ikeda, T. (2018). *Electronic fetal monitoring: The 5-tier system* (3rd ed.). Jones & Bartlett.

Pazos, R., Vuolo, K., Aladjem, S., Lueck, J., & Anderson, C. (1982). Association of spontaneous fetal heart rate decelerations during antepartum nonstress testing and intrauterine growth retardation. *American Journal of Obstetrics and Gynecology*, *144*(5), 574–577. https://doi.org/10 .1016/0002-9378(82)90230-7

Pearson, J., & Weaver, J. (1976). Fetal activity and fetal wellbeing: An evaluation. *British Medical Journal*, *1*(6021), 1305–1307. https://doi.org/10.1136/bmj.1.6021.1305

Perlman, J. M., & Risser, R. (1996). Can asphyxiated infants at risk for neonatal seizures be rapidly identified by current high-risk markers? *Pediatrics*, *97*(4), 456–462.

Perlman, J. M. (1997). Intrapartum hypoxic-ischemic cerebral injury and subsequent cerebral palsy: Medicolegal issues. *Pediatrics*, *99*(6), 851–859. https://doi.org/10.1542/peds.99.6.851

Pomerance, J. (1999). Umbilical cord blood gases casebook: Interpreting umbilical cord blood gases. *Journal of Perinatology*, *19*(8), 608–609. https://doi.org/10.1038/sj.jp.7200291

Pomerance, J. (2000). Umbilical cord blood gases casebook. Interpreting umbilical cord blood gases, VII. *Journal of Perinatology, 20*(5), 338–339. https://doi.org/10.1038/sj.jp.7200383

Reuwer, P. J., Bruinse, H. W., Stoutenbeek, P., & Haspels, A. A. (1984). Doppler assessment of the fetoplacental circulation in normal and growth-retarded fetuses. *European Journal of Obstetrics, Gynecology, and Reproductive Biology, 18*(4), 199–205. https://doi.org/10.1016/0028-2243(84)90117-5

Riley, R. J., & Johnson, J. W. (1993). Collecting and analyzing cord blood gases. *Clinical Obstetrics and Gynecology, 36*(1), 13–23. https://doi.org/10.1097/00003081-199303000-00005

Roberts, S., Leveno, K., Sidawai, J., Lucas, M., & Kelly, M. (1995). Fetal acidemia associated with regional anesthesia for elective cesarean delivery. *Obstetrics and Gynecology, 85*(1), 79–83. https://doi.org/10.1016/0029-7844(94)p4401-9

Ross, M. G., & Gala, R. (2002). Use of umbilical artery base excess: Algorithm for the timing of hypoxic injury. *American Journal of Obstetrics and Gynecology, 187*(1), 1–9. https://doi.org/10.1067/mob.2002.123204

Scheans, P. (2011). Umbilical cord blood gases: New clinical relevance for an age-old practice. *Neonatal Network, 30*(2), 123–126. https://doi.org/10.1891/0730-0832.30.2.123

Schwartz, N., & Young, N. (2006). Intrapartum fetal monitoring today. *Journal of Perinatal Medicine, 34*(2) 99–107.

Seeds, A. E. (1981). Basic concepts of maternal-fetal amniotic fluid exchange: Their relevance to fetal therapeutics. *Pediatric Clinics of North America, 28*, 231–240. https://doi.10.1016/s0031-3955(1)33973-6

Smith, C. V., Phelan, J. P., Platt, L. D., Broussard, P., & Paul, R. H. (1986). Fetal acoustic stimulation testing. II. A randomized clinical comparison with the nonstress test. *American Journal of Obstetrics and Gynecology, 155*(1), 131–134. https://doi.org/10.1016/0002-9378(86)90095-5

Tan, K. H., Smyth, R. M., & Wei, X. (2013). Fetal vibroacoustic stimulation for facilitation of tests of fetal wellbeing. *The Cochrane Database of Systematic Reviews,* (12), CD002963. https://doi.org/10.1002/14651858.CD002963.pub2

Tekin, A., Ozkan, S., Caliskan, E., Ozeren, S., Corakci, A., & Yucesoy, I. (2008). Fetal pulse oximetry: Correlation with intrapartum fetal heart rate patterns and neonatal outcome. *Journal of Obstetric and Gynaecologic Research, 34*(5), 824–831. https://doi.org/10.1111/j.1447-0756.2008.00850.x

Thompson, G., Newnham, J. P., Roberman, B. D., & Burns, S. E. (1990). Contraction stress fetal heart rate monitoring at preterm gestational ages. *The Australian & New Zealand Journal of Obstetrics & Gynaecology, 30*(2), 120–123. https://doi.org/10.1111/j.1479-828x.1990.tb03239.x

Thorp, J. A., Dildy, G. A., Yeomans, E. R., Meyer, B. A., & Parisi, V. M. (1996). Umbilical cord blood gas analysis at delivery. *American Journal of Obstetrics and Gynecology, 175*(3), 517–522. https://doi.org/10.1053/ob.1996.v175.a74401

Ullrich, J., & Ackerman, B. (1972). Changes in umbilical artery blood gas values with the onset of respiration. *Biology of the Neonate, 20*, 466–474. https://doi.org/10.1159/000240488

van den Berg, P. P., Nelen, W. L., Jongsma, H. W., Nijland, R., Kollée, L. A., Nijhuis, J. G., & Eskes, T. K. (1996). Neonatal complications in newborns with an umbilical artery pH < 7.00. *American Journal of Obstetrics and Gynecology, 175*(5), 1152–1157. https://doi.org/10.1016/s0002-9378(96)70021-2

Wallman, C. (1997). Interpretation of fetal cord blood gases. *Neonatal Network, 16*(1), 72–75.

White, C. R., Doherty, D. A., Henderson, J. J., Kohan, R., Newnham, J. P., & Pennell, C. E. (2010). Benefits of introducing universal umbilical cord blood gas and lactate analysis into an obstetric unit. *The Australian & New Zealand Journal of Obstetrics & Gynaecology, 50*(4), 318–328. https://doi.org/10.1111/j.1479-828X.2010.01192.x

Winkler, C. L., Hauth, J. C., Tucker, J. M., Owen, J., & Brumfield, C. G. (1991). Neonatal complications at term as related to the degree of umbilical artery acidemia. *American Journal of Obstetrics and Gynecology, 164*(2), 637–641. https://doi.org/10.1016/s0002-9378(11)80038-4

Wisner, K., & Holschuh, C. (2018). Fetal heart rate auscultation (3rd ed.). *Nursing for Women's Health, 22*(6), e1–e32. https://doi.org/10.1016/j.nwh.2018.10.001

Wu, Y. W., & Colford, J. M. (2000). Chorioamnionitis as a risk factor for cerebral palsy: A meta-analysis. *Journal of the American Medical Association, 284*(11), 1417–1424. https://doi.org/10.1001/jama.284.11.1417

Maternal, Fetal, and Placental Physiology

Antay L. Waters

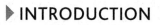

▶ INTRODUCTION

Fetal heart rate (FHR) patterns exhibit certain characteristics under the influence of hypoxic and nonhypoxic events. Clinicians should have a basic understanding of physiology of fetal respiratory exchange and FHR (Freeman et al., 2012). Electronic fetal monitoring (EFM) is a screening tool that allows clinicians ongoing observation of fetal physiology. Understanding the fetal oxygen pathway is the first step in the process of understanding the various intricate factors related to fetal oxygenation. The maternal respiratory system is the only source of oxygen for the fetus (Menihan & Kopel-Puretz, 2019). The oxygenation pathway moves from the environment → maternal lungs → maternal heart → maternal vasculature → maternal uterus → placenta → umbilical cord → fetus. Disruption of normal oxygen transfer can occur at any or all of the points along the oxygen pathway (Miller et al., 2017).

▶ OBJECTIVES

- Discuss factors involved in fetal oxygenation as they affect the oxygenation pathway.
- Review fetal circulation as it relates to fetal oxygenation.
- Understand the physiologic compensatory mechanisms available to the fetus in response to hypoxemia.
- Review the role of the placenta, including the various mechanisms for exchange.

▶ KEY TERMS

- **Aerobic Metabolism:** Occurring in the presence of oxygen; requiring oxygen for respiration. The chemical process of using oxygen to produce energy from carbohydrates
- **Anaerobic Metabolism:** Chemical process of energy production from carbohydrates that takes place in the absence of oxygen
- **Baroreceptors:** Pressure-sensitive stretch receptors in the carotid sinus and aortic arch that detect changes in blood pressure. Stimulation alters the FHR by stimulating the autonomic nervous system to increase or decrease the FHR via the sympathetic or parasympathetic branch
- **Chemoreceptors:** Sensory nerve endings or cells stimulated by increased or decreased blood concentration of a chemical. Sensitive to changes in oxygen, carbon dioxide, and pH levels in the blood. Located in the aortic and carotid bodies and in the medulla
- **Fetal Reserve:** Ability to maintain tissue oxygenation and essential physiologic functions in response to decreased oxygen availability
- **Medulla Oblongata:** Lower portion of the brainstem; relay center for the parasympathetic and sympathetic nervous systems
- **Parasympathetic Nervous System:** Part of the autonomic nervous system, including the vagus nerve (cranial nerve X); stimulation results in FHR decrease
- **Sympathetic Nervous System:** Part of the autonomic nervous system; stimulation results in FHR increase

▶ PHYSIOLOGY RELATED TO THE FETAL CIRCULATORY SYSTEM

Understanding the fetal cardiac system is imperative to understanding the physiology that affects fetal monitoring. Many factors interact to regulate FHR variability, including intrinsic cardiac pacemakers, cardiac conduction pathways, autonomic innervation (sympathetic and parasympathetic nervous systems), and intrinsic hormonal factors (catecholamines). The sinoatrial (SA) node serves as the physiologic primary pacemaker. Similar to adults, it is located in the right atrium and sets the rate in the normal heart. The atrioventricular (AV) node is the secondary pacemaker and is located in the atrial septum. The bundle of His and Purkinje fibers carry electrical signals throughout the ventricles at a slower rate than both the SA and the AV nodes. In a fetus, complete heart block is a rate between 60 and 80 bpm (Creasy et al., 2019).

In an adult, cardiac output (CO) is stroke volume (SV) × heart rate (HR). SV involves the stretching of the myocardium by an increased inflow of blood, causing the heart to contract with greater force and pump out more blood (also known as the Frank–Starling mechanism). Compared with adults, fetal SV does not fluctuate significantly. When more CO is required, the fetus compensates by increasing its HR, assuming it has a healthy heart and cardiac conduction system. The FHR is the product of many physiologic factors that modulate the intrinsic rate of the fetal heart. Factors that regulate the FHR include the autonomic nervous system (sympathetic and parasympathetic), which is the most common factor; the central nervous system (medulla oblongata, hypothalamus, and cerebral cortex); baroreceptors; chemoreceptors; and hormonal influences.

AUTONOMIC NERVOUS SYSTEM

The autonomic nervous system is one of the main biological systems that regulates physiology. Autonomic nervous system regulatory capacity begins before birth as the sympathetic and parasympathetic activity contributes significantly to fetal development. In the fetal stage, the heart and autonomic nerves develop simultaneously; however, the physiologic changes involving autonomic nervous activity that occur during the fetal stage have yet to be studied in detail. The autonomic nervous system is separated into sympathetic and parasympathetic:

- Sympathetic ("speedy")
  - Cardio-accelerator
- Parasympathetic ("pokey")
  - Cardio-decelerator
  - Constantly in conflict, causing FHR variability

Stimulation of the parasympathetic nervous system causes a decrease in the FHR and may trigger release of meconium. Release of meconium can be a normal physiologic response and does not necessarily indicate fetal compromise; however, it does place the neonate at risk if aspiration occurs.

Sympathetic Nervous System

The sympathetic nervous system matures earlier than the parasympathetic nervous system and is widely distributed within the cardiac muscle. Stimulation of sympathetic nerves releases norepinephrine, leading to increased FHR, increased strength of myocardial contraction, and increased CO secondary to increased FHR. This process is a reserve mechanism the fetus uses in stressful situations. The sympathetic nervous system is responsible for the increased release of norepinephrine, which increases firing of impulses. Sympathetic and parasympathetic responses both require oxygen to function maximally. They play a significant part in FHR variability. As a result, when the FHR baseline is stable and moderate variability and/or accelerations are present, it confirms the absence of both fetal metabolic acidemia and ongoing neurologic hypoxic injury at the time it is observed (Miller et al., 2017). It is important to remember that the opposite is not true; minimal or absent variability alone does not confirm the presence of fetal metabolic acidemia or ongoing hypoxic injury (Miller et al., 2017).

Parasympathetic Nervous System

The parasympathetic nervous system controls the fetal heart via the vagus nerve (cranial nerve X), which originates in the medulla oblongata. The vagus nerve fibers innervate both the SA and the AV nodes of the heart and mature at around 26 to 28 weeks' gestation. Stimulation of the vagus nerve causes the release of acetylcholine at the myoneural synapse and decreases the firing of the SA node as well as the FHR. The vagus nerve also influences variability. Parasympathetic stimulation appears to have a greater influence than sympathetic regulation on the transmission of FHR variability. Vagal tone naturally increases with increasing gestational age, causing the FHR baseline to lower with increasing fetal maturity (Creasy et al., 2019).

CENTRAL NERVOUS SYSTEM

One of the most important components of the central nervous system related to regulation of the FHR is the cerebral cortex, which responds to fetal movement, increases or decreases reactivity and variability, and controls the fetal sleep center. With increasing gestational age, fetal sleep–wake cycles become more distinct. The fetal cerebellum is responsible for motor coordination as well as higher cognitive processes such as executive control related to language and social emotion. Another vital part of the central nervous system involves chemoreceptors and baroreceptors, whose goals include maintaining homeostasis by indirectly altering the FHR, AV conduction, and peripheral vascular resistance. They form a feedback loop that increases and decreases the FHR (King & Parer, 2000).

Baroreceptors

Baroreceptors are stretch receptors located in the aortic arch and carotid sinus. They sense pressure changes in the vessel walls (Menihan & Kopel-Puretz, 2019). Baroreceptors are related to blood pressure with the goal of maintaining homeostasis. In adults, the higher centers of the brain influence the HR, which is increased by emotional stimuli, such as when fear is experienced. A rise in blood pressure causes vagal stimulation, leading to reflex bradycardia, decrease in CO, and decrease in blood pressure that protect the fetus from the effects of excessive arterial pressure. A fall in fetal arterial blood pressure causes baroreceptors to receive less stimulation, leading to a reflex increase in the FHR.

Chemoreceptors

The primary function of chemoreceptors is regulation of respiratory activity and control of circulation by responding to changes in arterial partial pressure of oxygen (pO_2), partial pressure of carbon dioxide (pCO_2), and acid-base balance in the blood or cerebrospinal fluid. Chemoreceptors are nerve receptors found in both peripheral and central nervous system blood vessels that sense the chemical makeup of the surrounding environment. They are slower in response than baroreceptors. A change in the pH of the blood can cause an initiation to either increase or decrease the HR (Menihan & Kopel-Puretz, 2019). Chemoreceptors are related to oxygen and chemicals with the goal of maintaining homeostasis.

There are two types of chemoreceptors: peripheral and central. Peripheral chemoreceptors are located in the aortic arch and carotid bodies. Central chemoreceptors are located in the medulla oblongata. Both types are better understood in adults. When arterial blood perfusing the central chemoreceptors in the adult contain increased pCO_2 or decreased pO_2, reflex tachycardia and hypertension occur in an attempt to circulate the blood and rid the body of excessive pCO_2. Interaction of central and peripheral chemoreceptors in the fetus is not well understood. In the fetus, when arterial blood perfusing the central chemoreceptors contains increased pCO_2 or decreased pO_2, bradycardia results.

HORMONAL INFLUENCES

The adrenal medulla responds to stressful stimuli by producing epinephrine, norepinephrine, and a sympathetic response. In response, the FHR and blood pressure increase and greater force of contraction of the fetal heart occurs. The adrenal cortex maintains homeostasis related to blood volume. A low fetal blood pressure stimulates the release of aldosterone leading to decreased sodium output, increased water retention, and increased circulating blood volume. Arginine vasopressin is a plasma catecholamine secreted by the pituitary gland. In the fetus, it is the most potent stimulus released during periods of hypoxemia as well as during hemorrhage. It also serves to help regulate fetal blood pressure, produces a rise in blood pressure by increasing peripheral vascular resistance, and decreases the FHR. It also causes decreased blood flow to nonvital organs.

Renin-angiotensin II in the adult is released by adrenals when there is a decrease in plasma volume or blood pressure, stimulating vasoconstriction to maintain blood pressure. In the fetus, angiotensin II and aldosterone levels do not increase in proportion to changes in plasma renin (in contrast to the neonate and the adult). Uncoupling of the fetal renin–angiotensin–aldosterone system is due to many factors and is likely to protect the fetus from hemorrhagic stress by stimulating vasoconstriction (Creasy et al., 2019). Angiotensin II may play a role in fetal circulatory regulation at rest. The majority of its activity is observed during hemorrhagic stress on the fetus (Creasy et al., 2019). A variety of prostaglandins are found in the fetal blood and tissue with the main function of regulating umbilical blood flow and the patency of the ductus arteriosus during fetal life.

FETAL CIRCULATION

The fetal circulation system (Figure 3.1) is distinctly different from the adult circulation system. This intricate system allows the fetus to receive oxygenated blood and nutrients from the placenta. Fetal circulation bypasses the lungs via a shunt known as the ductus arteriosus; the liver is also bypassed via the ductus venosus, and blood can travel from the right atrium to the left atrium via the foramen ovale. When compared with adults, fetuses have decreased ventricular filling and reduced contractility; however, fetal CO is higher per unit of weight than in an adult. The fetus also has more capillaries per unit of tissue than adults (Finnemore & Groves, 2015). The fetal heart begins beating approximately 22 days after fertilization, marking the initiation of fetal circulation. Gas exchange initially occurs in the yolk sac until the placenta entirely takes over. This transition occurs at around 10 weeks' gestation. Maternal oxygenated blood mixes with placental blood, which is low in oxygen, before heading out to the fetus. Due to this mixing, the fetus is relatively hypoxic compared to maternal arterial blood (Morton & Brodsky, 2016). At delivery, the neonatal cardiovascular system undergoes a quick, drastic

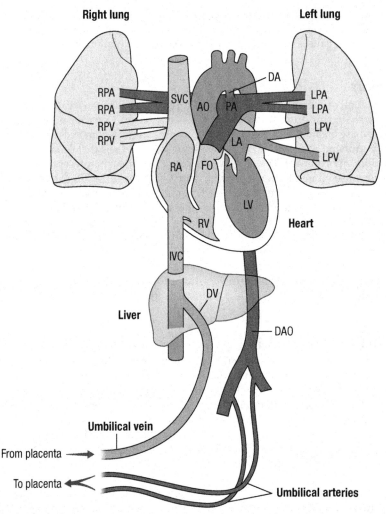

Figure 3.1 Fetal circulation.

AO, aorta; DA, ductus arteriosus; DAO, descending aorta; DV, ductus venosus; FO, foramen ovale; IVC, interior vena cava; LA, left atrium; LPA, left pulmonary artery; LPV, left pulmonary vein; LV, left ventricle; PA, pulmonary artery; RA, right atrium; RPA, right pulmonary artery; RPV, right pulmonary vein; RV, right ventricle; SVC, superior vena cava.

Source: Bellini, S., & Beaulieu, M. (2017). *Neonatal advanced practice nursing: A case-based learning approach.* Springer Publishing Company.

change. With its first breath, the neonate's pulmonary vascular resistance substantially drops in response to the oxygen now present in the lungs and the physical act of breathing. With the umbilical cord clamping after birth, the systemic vascular resistance increases, helping the blood flow toward the lungs. The ductus arteriosus has a left-to-right flow within 10 minutes. The smooth muscle in the ductus arteriosus responds to the oxygen by increasing calcium channel activity, causing constriction and ultimately shunt closure. The increased systemic resistance also raises the pressure in the left atrium to be higher than that in the right atrium, and this causes the foramen ovale to close (Morton & Brodsky, 2016).

The placenta connects the maternal and fetal circulatory systems, providing oxygen and nutrients from the pregnant patient to the growing fetus. It also removes metabolic wastes and carbon dioxide from the fetus via the blood vessels in the umbilical cord. Oxygenated blood in the placenta flows through the umbilical vein to be distributed partially to the fetal hepatic circulation but mostly into the inferior vena cava (IVC), bypassing the liver via the ductus venosus, with an estimated oxygen saturation of 70% to 80%—the highest concentration of oxygen-rich blood supply to the fetus. From the IVC, blood travels through the right atrium. There is greater pressure in the right atrium compared with the left atrium in fetal circulation; therefore, most of the oxygenated blood is shunted from the right atrium to the left atrium through the foramen ovale, whereas a mixture of oxygenated blood from the IVC and deoxygenated blood from the superior vena cava becomes partially oxygenated blood in the right atrium. As a result, the estimated oxygen saturation of the left atrium is 65% compared with the right atrium, which is only 55%. Once the oxygenated blood reaches the left atrium, it travels through the left ventricle into the coronary arteries and the aorta, which branches to provide the most oxygenated blood to the brain before a shunt from the pulmonary artery—the ductus arteriosus—allows partially oxygenated blood to be combined with the blood supply that will then flow to the systemic circulation with an estimated oxygen saturation of 60%. The partially oxygenated blood in the right atrium, as mentioned previously, can also enter the right ventricle and then the pulmonary artery. Because there is high resistance to blood flow in the lungs, the blood is shunted from the pulmonary artery into the aorta via the ductus arteriosus, mostly bypassing the lungs. Blood then enters the systemic circulation, and the deoxygenated blood, with an estimated oxygen saturation of 40%, is recycled back to the placenta via the umbilical arteries to be oxygenated again by the pregnant patient (Morton & Brodsky, 2016).

Clinical Pearl

Comprehensive understanding of fetal circulation is imperative for complete understanding of FHR physiology.

FETAL SLEEP–WAKE CYCLES

It is important to note that the FHR is also affected by fetal sleep–wake cycles, which begin to become more apparent during the third trimester. The two most common fetal states during the third trimester are quiet sleep and active (REM) sleep. The average time spent during a fetal sleep cycle, or quiet state, is approximately 16 minutes per hour; however, it can last up to 20 to 40 minutes in a term fetus. The number of FHR accelerations per hour during active states increases with advanced gestational age (Suwanrath & Suntharasaj, 2010). While a fetus may maintain moderate variability during a sleep cycle, it is not uncommon to see only minimal variability.

▶ PHYSIOLOGY OF THE OXYGEN PATHWAY

MATERNAL BLOOD FLOW

Maternal blood travels to the pulmonary alveoli, where 98% of oxygen combines with hemoglobin in red blood cells. Approximately 1% to 2% of oxygen dissolves in the blood and is measured by the partial pressure of dissolved oxygen (PaO_2). The amount of oxygen that remains bound to hemoglobin depends on the normal adult PaO_2 of 95 to 100 mmHg, resulting in a hemoglobin saturation of approximately 95% to 98%. This means that the maternal hemoglobin is carrying 95% to 98% of the total oxygen that it is able to support (Menihan & Kopel-Puretz, 2019). Adequate fetal oxygenation is dependent on adequate maternal oxygenation.

As a result of pregnancy, remodeling occurs involving the structure and function of the uterine arteries and veins. The arteries change from tightly coiled, high-pressure vessels to dilated vessels in order to accommodate large blood volumes and decrease peripheral resistance (King & Parer, 2000). If the remodeling process is impeded during placental growth, the spiral arteries remain tightly coiled. In pregnancy, the arteries lose their ability to autoregulate (the vessels do not constrict to allow for increased blood flow if the pressure in the vessels drops). This means that the volume of blood delivered to the intervillous space is dependent on adequate blood flow to the uterus.

The maternal blood supply to the uterus is via the uterine and ovarian arteries that form the arcuate arteries and from which radial arteries penetrate the myometrium. The radial arteries then divide into spiral arteries that supply the intervillous space, bathing the chorionic villi in maternal blood. The pressure is about 80 to 100 mmHg in the uterine arteries, 70 mmHg in the spiral arteries, and only 10 mmHg within the intervillous space (Griffiths & Campbell, 2015). It is important to note that no pharmacologic agents can increase vasodilatation in the uteroplacental unit; however, increased blood flow to the uterus can occur through maternal position changes, by maintaining maternal blood pressure, and with tocolytics in the presence of tachysystole. Blood supply in the intervillous space is maximized when the patient is resting in the lateral position as compared with the supine position (Freeman et al., 2012).

PLACENTA

The placenta is an endocrine organ that produces both steroids (estrogen and progesterone) and protein (human gonadotropin hormone and human placental lactogen) and serves as the fetal lungs, kidneys, and gastrointestinal tract and as a barrier to certain dangerous substances. Uteroplacental circulation is not fully established until the end of the first trimester. The exact mechanism of how the uteroplacental circulation is established is not completely understood. Uterine perfusion accounts for 10% to 15% of maternal CO (approximately 700–800 mL/min). Uterine blood flow is supplied from the uterine arteries. The spiral arteries must traverse through the thickness of the myometrium to reach the intervillous space. Approximately 85% of total uterine blood flow supplies the placental (intervillous) circulation. If blood flow to any area of the intervillous space is compromised, a placental infarct may occur. The remaining 15% supplies the extraplacental uterine musculature. Maternal blood occupies the intervillous space where maternal and fetal blood exchange. The placenta is referred to as a hemochorial type because maternal blood comes in direct contact with fetal blood. Anything that affects maternal CO will affect the flow of blood through the spiral arteries. As the uterus contracts, the intramyometrial pressure may exceed the intraarterial pressure, causing an occlusion of these vessels and cessation of blood flow (Griffiths & Campbell, 2014).

> ### Clinical Pearl
>
> Maternal repositioning, particularly in the lateral position, is crucial to improving placental blood flow.

Factors That Decrease Placental Blood Flow

Multiple factors can decrease placental blood flow, including:

- Changes in maternal position, primarily supine due to uterine compression of the IVC and aortoiliac vessels.
- Exercise diverting blood away from the uterus to supply oxygen to maternal muscles, which results in decreased uterine blood flow. FHR is increased (tachycardia possible) due to a sympathetic response to reduced fetal oxygenation or hypoxia. The fetus is affected only with *excessive* exercise.
- Tachysystole—however, if uterine oxygen exchange is normal, contractions do not compromise the fetus.
- Anything affecting the surface area of the placenta will compromise fetal oxygenation, such as a placental abruption or the premature separation of the placenta from the uterine wall.
- Analgesia and anesthesia may produce both therapeutic and side effects, potentially altering maternal and fetal assessments. Reassessment and documentation of efficacy and side effects as well as fetal status should occur within 30 to 60 minutes of such interventions:

- Maternal hypotension reduces intervillous space blood flow. If position changes and IV fluid bolus are not successful, administration of either IV ephedrine or IV phenylephrine may be needed.
- The American Society of Anesthesiologists recommends considering phenylephrine to improve fetal acid-base status if no maternal bradycardia is present. Ephedrine is associated with fetal acidosis due to placental transfer and direct fetal metabolism (Lim et al., 2018).
- Maternal hypertension decreases intervillous space flow due to acute or chronic changes.
- Diffusion distance because the thickness of the placental membrane between the intervillous space and the fetal capillaries may decrease transfer of oxygen:
  - Villous hemorrhage and edema in the diabetic patient may play a role in placental thickness.
- Vasa previa is typically diagnosed during pregnancy; however, it is imperative that clinicians be able to recognize an undiagnosed vasa previa. Signs and symptoms include:
  - Painless vaginal bleeding at time of rupture of membranes.
  - Fetal shock and/or demise (can occur rapidly).
  - Before rupture of membranes (ROM), possible cord compression EFM pattern.
  - Possible ability to palpate vessels on vaginal exam.

Placental Exchange

The fetal lungs do not take part in gas exchange while in utero, so the placenta is wholly responsible for the transfer of oxygen and carbon dioxide to and from the developing fetus. Oxygen is a small molecule that readily crosses the placenta by passive diffusion. Oxygen transfer mainly depends on the oxygen partial pressure gradient between maternal blood in the intervillous space and fetal blood in the umbilical arteries. Oxygen transfer to the fetus is enhanced by the Bohr effect. At the maternal-fetal interface, maternal blood takes up carbon dioxide and becomes more acidotic. This causes a rightward shift of the maternal oxyhemoglobin dissociation curve, which favors oxygen release to the fetus. At the same time, fetal blood releases carbon dioxide and becomes more alkalotic (Mushambi et al., 2002). Carbon dioxide also crosses the placenta readily by passive diffusion. Transfer from the fetus to the pregnant patient depends mainly on the partial pressure gradient for carbon dioxide between fetal blood in the umbilical arteries and maternal blood in the intervillous space. Carbon dioxide transfer from the fetus to the pregnant patient is facilitated by the Haldane effect (the increased capacity of deoxygenated blood to carry carbon dioxide compared with oxygenated blood). As maternal blood releases oxygen (producing deoxyhemoglobin), it is able to carry more carbon dioxide as bicarbonate and carbaminohemoglobin. At the same time, as fetal blood takes up oxygen to form oxyhemoglobin, it has reduced affinity for carbon dioxide and therefore releases carbon dioxide to the patient (Mushambi et al., 2002).

The fetus has very little capacity for gluconeogenesis, so maternal glucose forms its main source of energy. Passive diffusion of glucose across the placenta is insufficient to meet the needs of the fetus, and therefore facilitated diffusion using a variety of glucose transporters is required. Amino acids for fetal protein synthesis are transferred from the patient to fetus by active transport. There are several transporter proteins specific for anionic, cationic, and neutral amino acids. Many of these proteins concurrently transport amino acids with sodium: the transport of sodium down its concentration gradient drags amino acids into the cells. Fatty acids are important for the synthesis of compounds involved in cell signaling (prostaglandins and leukotrienes) and for the production of fetal phospholipids, biological membranes, and myelin. Free fatty acids and glycerol are transferred from patient to fetus mainly by simple diffusion but also through the use of fatty acid binding proteins (Desforges & Sibley, 2009; Knipp et al., 1999). Sodium and chloride ions are mainly transferred across the placenta by passive diffusion, although active transport may have a role. Calcium ions, iron, and vitamins are transferred by active carrier-mediated transport. Water moves by simple diffusion according to hydrostatic and osmotic pressure gradients. Certain water channel proteins in the trophoblast may aid its passage (Gude et al., 2004).

Almost all drugs will eventually cross the placenta to reach the fetus. In some cases, this transplacental transfer may be beneficial, and drugs may be deliberately administered to the pregnant patient to treat specific fetal conditions. For example, steroids may be given to the patient to promote fetal lung maturation, and cardiac drugs may be given to control fetal arrhythmias. However, the transplacental passage of drugs may also have detrimental effects on the fetus, including teratogenicity or impairment of fetal growth and development. The greatest risk of adverse drug effects on the fetus is probably during organogenesis. The effects of drugs on the fetus either may be direct or may be mediated via the alteration of uteroplacental blood flow. Three types of drug transfer across the placenta are recognized:

■ Complete transfer (type 1 drugs): Drugs exhibiting this type of transfer will rapidly cross the placenta with pharmacologically significant concentrations equilibrating in maternal and fetal blood, such as thiopental and propofol.
■ Exceeding transfer (type 2 drugs): These drugs cross the placenta to reach greater concentrations in fetal compared with maternal blood, such as ketamine.
■ Incomplete transfer (type 3 drugs): These drugs are unable to cross the placenta completely, resulting in higher concentrations in maternal blood compared with fetal blood, such as succinylcholine or insulin (Griffiths & Campbell, 2015).

Drugs that transfer from the maternal to the fetal blood must be carried into the intervillous space and pass through the syncytiotrophoblast, fetal connective tissue, and endothelium of fetal capillaries. The rate-limiting barrier for placental drug transfer is the layer of syncytiotrophoblast cells covering the villi.
There are four main mechanisms of drug transfer across the placenta:

1. **Simple/passive diffusion**—Most drugs cross the placenta by this mechanism. Transfer is either transcellularly through the syncytiotrophoblast layer or paracellularly through water channels incorporated into the membrane. Diffusion does not require energy input but is dependent on a concentration gradient across the placenta with drug passively moving from areas of high to low concentration (Audus, 1999).
2. **Facilitated diffusion**—Drugs structurally related to endogenous compounds are often transported by facilitated diffusion. This type of transport needs a carrier substance within the placenta to facilitate transfer across it. Again, energy input is not required since drug transfer occurs down a concentration gradient. Facilitated diffusion will be inhibited if the carrier molecules become saturated by both drug and endogenous substrates competing for their use (Pacifici & Nottoli, 1995).
3. **Active transport**—Active transport uses energy, usually in the form of adenosine triphosphate (ATP), to transport substances against a concentration or electrochemical gradient. Transport is carrier-mediated and saturable, and there is competition between related molecules. Active drug transporters are located on both the maternal and the fetal sides of the placental membranes and can transport drugs from patient to fetus and vice versa (Eshkoli et al., 2011).
4. **Pinocytosis**—Drugs become completely enveloped into invaginations of the membrane and are then released on the other side of the cell. Very little is known about this method of transfer and about the drugs that cross the placenta by this mechanism.

OXYGEN TRANSPORT

Fetal homeostatic mechanisms all interact and influence blood flow to promote oxygenation and protect vital organs. These mechanisms provide for reflex responses to both nonhypoxemic and hypoxemic stress. The fetal ability to extract oxygen is greater than that of the pregnant patient. Fetal hemoglobin also has a higher affinity for oxygen and a higher concentration, resulting in the fetus having an added ability to carry more oxygen. The normal, healthy fetus can withstand repeated transient hypoxemia from uterine contractions and can maintain normal aerobic metabolism until oxygen in the intervillous space falls to 50% of normal levels (King & Parer, 2000). When pO_2 falls significantly, fetal circulatory responses to hypoxia include:

■ Redistribution of blood flow favoring vital organs: brain, heart, and adrenal glands
■ Loss of cerebral vascular autoregulation resulting in a pressure-passive cerebral circulation
■ An eventual decrease in fetal myocardial oxygen consumption resulting in hypotension and ultimately a decrease in cerebral blood flow

Noncirculatory responses to hypoxia include:

■ Slower depletion of high-energy compounds during hypoxic events
■ Use of alternative energy substrates, such as lactic acid and ketone bodies, and anaerobic metabolism in certain vascular beds
■ Resistance of the fetal and neonatal myocardium to hypoxic events
■ Potential protractive role of fetal hemoglobin

Because of these circulatory and noncirculatory responses to hypoxia, the fetus has considerable protection from neuronal damage. Prolonged or repeated hypoxemia or a lack of fetal reserves before labor may deplete fetal resources and result in decompensation (King & Parer, 2000). Deterioration in fetal oxygenation may occur when there is a disruption at any point in the oxygen pathway (Box 3.1).

Box 3.1: Fetal Cascade of Deterioration During Disrupted Oxygenation

---

Hypoxemia → Low levels of oxygen in the blood. If recurrent or sustained, leads to hypoxia.

↓

Hypoxia → Decreased delivery of oxygen to tissues with levels inadequate to meet metabolic needs. If hypoxemia/hypoxia progress and the fetal oxygen reserves are used, the fetus moves into anaerobic metabolism.

↓

Anaerobic metabolism → Decreased cardiac muscle effectiveness, decreased functionality and coordination of the autonomic nervous system. As a result, lactic acid accumulates and metabolic acidosis results.

↓

Acidosis → Abnormal excess hydrogen ion concentration in tissues due to the acid accumulation or base consumption; lactic acid transfers slowly across the placenta. Buffer bases (primarily sodium bicarbonate [HCO_3]) are used in an effort to neutralize the lactic acid. If buffer bases are depleted, the blood pH may fall, leading to metabolic acidemia.

↓

Acidemia → Abnormal excess hydrogen ion concentration in the blood due to the acid accumulation or base consumption. The more hydrogen ions are present, the more acidic the blood and lower the pH. If tissue hypoxia and acidosis are recurrent or sustained, loss of peripheral vascular smooth muscle contraction and reduced peripheral vascular resistance will lead to fetal hypotension.

↓

Fetal hypotension → Fetus is at risk for cellular damage and injury, typically with umbilical artery pH <7.0 and base deficit >12 mmol/L

AMNIOTIC FLUID

Amniotic fluid surrounds the embryo and fetus during development and has many functions. Physically, it protects the fetus in the event the maternal abdomen is subjected to trauma. It also protects the umbilical cord by providing a cushion between the fetus and the umbilical cord, thus reducing the risk of compression between the fetus and the uterine wall. Amniotic fluid also helps protect the fetus from infectious agents due to its inherent antibacterial properties. Additionally, it serves as a reservoir of fluid and nutrients for the fetus, containing proteins, electrolytes, immunoglobulins, and vitamins from the pregnant patient. It provides the necessary fluid, space, and growth factors to allow normal development and growth of fetal organs such as the musculoskeletal, gastrointestinal, and pulmonary systems (Tong et al., 2009). Clinicians can also use amniotic fluid as a tool to monitor the progression of pregnancy and predict fetal outcomes.

The development of amniotic fluid organizes into early gestation and late gestation. Early gestation is the embryonic period, which is from the start of fertilization to 8 weeks, and late gestation encompasses the fetal period from 8 weeks to birth. The composition of amniotic fluid changes from early gestation to late gestation. During the embryonic period, amniotic fluid derives from both fetal and maternal factors, such as water from maternal serum, coelomic fluid, and fluid from the amniotic cavity; however, during late gestation, amniotic fluid is largely produced by fetal urine and lung secretions (Beall et al., 2007; Suliburska et al., 2016). The amount of amniotic fluid is greatest at about 4 weeks' gestation, when it averages 800 mL. About 600 mL of amniotic fluid surrounds the fetus at term.

Abnormally high or low amniotic fluid volumes have been shown to predict poor fetal outcomes; therefore, a normal amount of amniotic fluid volume is crucial to the healthy development of the fetus or embryo. Amniotic fluid has proven to be a major diagnostic tool when monitoring the progression and health of a pregnancy. Clinicians can use the amniotic fluid index (AFI) or maximum vertical pocket (MVP; Campbell et al., 1992; Kornacki et al., 2017). These measurements are part of the biophysical profile that consists of fetal tone, fetal movement, fetal breathing, and a nonstress test. AFI and single deepest pocket (SDP) or MVP are estimations of amniotic fluid volume based on ultrasound measurements. An AFI ≥24 cm or an MVP ≥8 cm is considered polyhydramnios. Polyhydramnios can be caused by maternal diabetes, gastrointestinal tract obstruction, genetic disorders, musculoskeletal disorders, or congenital diaphragmatic hernias. Conversely, oligohydramnios is an AFI ≤5 cm or an MVP ≤2 cm. Oligohydramnios can cause complications such as maternal diabetes, hypertensive disorders of pregnancy, renal agenesis, genitourinary tract obstruction, intrauterine growth restriction, or any condition that leads to placental insufficiency (Kehl et al., 2016; Moore, 2011). Amniotic fluid remains a vital substance required for the embryo or fetus to survive and helps clinicians make decisions regarding care and predict outcomes.

▶ ANATOMY AND PHYSIOLOGY OF THE UMBILICAL CORD

The umbilical cord allows for the transfer of oxygen and nutrients from maternal circulation into fetal circulation while simultaneously removing waste products from fetal circulation to be eliminated maternally. The umbilical cord is a bundle of blood vessels that develops during the early stages of embryologic development; it is enclosed inside a tubular sheath of amnion and consists of two paired umbilical arteries and one umbilical vein. During development, the umbilical arteries have a vital function of carrying deoxygenated blood away from the fetus to the placenta (Barrios-Arpi et al., 2017). However, after birth, a significant distal portion of the umbilical artery degenerates. These remnants later obliterate, forming the medial umbilical ligament. At the same time, the proximal portion of each umbilical artery serves as a branching point for the development of the anterior internal iliac arteries. The internal iliac arteries later give rise to the superior vesical arteries that supply the urinary bladder and ureters, as well as the ductus deferens and seminal vesicles in males (Hooper et al., 2015; Mamatha et al., 2015). The umbilical cord is a vital structure for the entire period of development because it tethers the fetus to the placenta and the uterine wall while also acting as the primary route to enable blood to circulate between the fetus and the placenta. The umbilical cord is a soft, tortuous cord with a smooth outer covering of amnion. It extends from the umbilicus of the fetus to the center of the placenta. Its length ranges from 50 to 60 cm with a diameter of about 1 cm. The umbilical cord is composed of a gelatinous substance called Wharton's jelly, which provides protection and insulation for the umbilical vessels. It also encloses the urachus, a fibrous remnant of the allantois that extends through the umbilical cord and is located in the space of Retzius between the peritoneum posteriorly and the transverse fascia anteriorly. The urachus serves as a drainage canal for the fetal urinary bladder.

The umbilical arteries carry deoxygenated blood from fetal circulation to the placenta. The two umbilical arteries converge at about 5 mm from the insertion of the cord, forming a type of vascular connection called the Hyrtl's anastomosis (Ullberg et al., 2001). The primary function of Hyrtl's anastomosis is to equalize blood flow and pressure between the umbilical and placental arteries (Ullberg et al., 2001). As the arteries enter the placenta, each bifurcates into smaller branches called the chorionic vessels. The thin-walled umbilical vein carries oxygenated blood and nutrients from the placenta to the fetus and is easily compressed.

PHYSIOLOGIC VARIANTS

False Knots in the Umbilical Cord

False knots are bulging masses located on the surface of the umbilical cord. Sometimes, excessive torsion of the umbilical cord inside the uterus can cause these bulging masses to appear as knots on uterine ultrasonography. The "knot" appearance of this condition forms via the excessive accumulation of Wharton's jelly bulks alternating with areas with relatively less jelly appearing as constrictions after each bulging. Hence, they are identified as false knots of the umbilical cord. This physiologic variation does not affect the stability of the fetal position, nor does it affect umbilical blood flow and pressure. Thus, false knots do not represent a considerable risk to the fetus (Feliks & Howorka, 1968).

Single Umbilical Artery

The incidence of having a single umbilical artery is very low overall; however, it is believed to be more common in multiparous patients than in nulliparous ones. Many studies have reported that the left umbilical artery is more often absent than the right (Lubusky et al., 2007). The side of umbilical artery absence has very minimal significance, with the exception of one study that concluded that infants with a single umbilical artery identified by ultrasound in utero had the presence of congenital abnormalities, including cardiac, renal, intestinal, and skeletal anomalies when the left umbilical artery was absent (Abuhamad et al., 1995; Blazer et al., 1997; Budorick et al., 2001; Geipel et al., 2000; Lubusky et al., 2007).

CLINICAL SIGNIFICANCE OF VARIOUS UMBILICAL CORD ANOMALIES

Velamentous Insertion

The incidence of velamentous insertion of the umbilical cord is significantly higher for in vitro fertilization (IVF)–induced pregnancies compared with naturally conceived pregnancies. It happens in about 10% of pregnancies and 20% of IVF pregnancies (Shevell et al., 2005). Velamentous insertion of the umbilical cord occurs when the placental end of the umbilical cord consists of umbilical arteries and veins surrounded by fetal membranes without Wharton's jelly. The exact reason for this condition is still unclear; however, the most current hypothesis suggests that during IVF pregnancy, half of the placenta undergoes excessive proliferation, causing the site of the insertion of the umbilical cord to move peripherally away from its center. Conversely, the other pole of the placenta involutes, and the umbilical cord becomes unable to follow the migration of the placenta (Yanaihara et al., 2018).

Four-Vessel Umbilical Cord

Normal umbilical cord anatomy consists of three vessels—two umbilical arteries and one umbilical vein. By the seventh week of gestation, the right umbilical vein usually obliterates, leaving a single (left) umbilical vein patent. However, there have been documented cases of umbilical cords containing four vessels. The persistence of two umbilical veins and two umbilical arteries within the umbilical cord is associated with multiple cardiovascular and gastrointestinal anomalies (Painter & Russell, 1977). When both the right and the left umbilical veins remain open, a condition called persistent right umbilical vein occurs, typically due to a deficiency in folic acid during the first trimester of pregnancy. This condition may cause teratogenic effects for the fetus and act as a risk factor for its overall physical health (Kim et al., 2018).

True Knots of the Umbilical Cord

True knots are real tangling nodules of the umbilical vessels along the length of the umbilical cord. They usually occur early in pregnancy as a result of various predisposing factors. Most commonly, the development of true knots is associated with the presence of excessive amniotic fluid, causing high pressure on the umbilical cord vessels and increasing their torsional force, causing deep knots of those vessels. Also, an increase in the movement of the fetus in utero plays a vital role in creating that teratogenic deformity, as supercoils of the umbilical cord can cause it to knot over itself. True knot deformities of the umbilical cord are very dangerous because they may obstruct blood flow in the umbilical vessels, which may eventually lead to fetal demise (Sepulveda et al., 1995).

Very Short Umbilical Cord

An umbilical cord is considered significantly short when its length is less than approximately 40 cm. A short umbilical cord can lead to cord avulsion, resulting in an interruption in fetal circulation, causing intrauterine bleeding followed by fetal death (Olaya-C & Bernal, 2015).

Very Long Umbilical Cord

If an umbilical cord is longer than 65 to 70 cm, it is clinically considered long. An abnormally long umbilical cord has greater potential to lead to a nuchal cord with multiple loops around the fetal neck, contributing to fetal hypoxia and possible death, as well as increased risk for umbilical cord prolapse (Olaya-C & Bernal, 2015).

▶ KEY POINTS

- ■ Evaluation of EFM should be done with the understanding of fetal sleep–wake cycles, particularly during the third trimester, to prevent unnecessary interventions.
- ■ A strong understanding of the physiology of fetal circulation and changes at the time of delivery is imperative for any clinician caring for patients at the time of delivery.

■ The placenta's interrelationship between the pregnant patient and the fetus in the delivery of oxygen and nutrients and the removal of waste is paramount. Fetal health and growth are dependent on this complex interaction.

CASE STUDY

Elizabeth is a 33-year-old G2P0010 patient at 38 weeks and 3 days' gestation admitted to labor and delivery for induction of labor for chronic hypertension with superimposed preeclampsia without severe features. Sterile vaginal exam on admission is 1/25/-3 with intact amniotic membranes. Induction is started with insertion of a Cook balloon and oxytocin (Pitocin). The following EFM tracing is obtained approximately 4 hours after oxytocin (Pitocin) initiation.

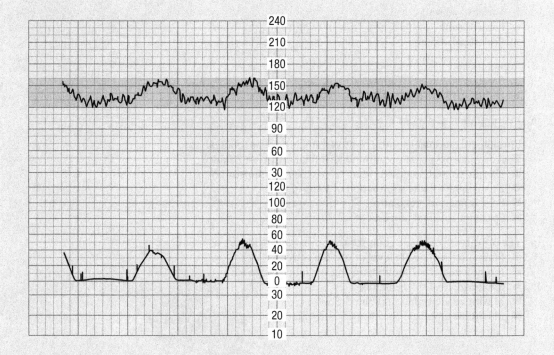

Answer the following questions, and then see "Case Study Answers" for the correct answers.

1. Baseline FHR: _____

2. Variability: _____

3. Accelerations: Present or absent?

4. Decelerations:
   a. Early: Present or absent?
   b. Variable: Present or absent?
   c. Late: Present or absent?
   d. Prolonged: Present or absent?

5. Contractions:
   a. Frequency: _____
   b. Duration: _____

6. Interpretation: Category _____

7. List all possible physiologic rationales for the observed tracing.

8. List, in order, the priority physiologic goals for the observed tracing.

(See answers next page.)

CASE STUDY ANSWERS

1. Baseline FHR: 130 bpm

2. Variability: Moderate

3. Accelerations: Present

4. Decelerations:
   a. Early: Absent
   b. Variable: Absent
   c. Late: Absent
   d. Prolonged: Absent

5. Contractions
   a. Frequency: Every 2 minutes
   b. Duration: 50 to 60 seconds

6. Interpretation: Category I

7. Physiologic rationales for the observed tracing are as follows:
   - Adequate oxygenation with normal fetal acid-base balance
   - Uterine contractions secondary to oxytocin administration
   - Direct sympathetic stimulation of fetus
   - Fetal autonomic regulation
   - Spontaneous fetal movement

8. The priority physiologic goals for the observed tracing are as follows:
   - Maintain appropriate level of uterine activity.
   - Promote maternal comfort during the labor process.
   - Maximize fetal oxygenation.
   - Maximize uteroplacental blood flow.
   - Maximize umbilical cord flow.

● KNOWLEDGE CHECK: CHAPTER 3

1. The vagus nerve matures between 26 and 28 weeks. Its dominance results in what effect to the fetal heart rate (FHR) baseline?
   A. Decrease
   B. Increase
   C. No change

2. The fetus compensates for decreased maternal circulating volume by increasing cardiac output (CO) by increasing:
   A. Fetal movement
   B. Heart rate (HR)
   C. Stroke volume (SV)

3. The fetal heart rate (FHR) is controlled by the:
   A. Atrioventricular (AV) node
   B. Sinoatrial (SA) node
   C. Sympathetic nervous system

4. Well-oxygenated blood enters the fetal heart directly, bypassing the liver, via the:
   A. Ductus arteriosus
   B. Ductus venosus
   C. Foramen ovale

5. Compared with maternal blood, oxygen affinity in fetal blood has:
   A. Easier release of oxygen to tissues
   B. Greater binding of oxygen
   C. Greater stimulation of erythropoietin release

6. Baroreceptors respond mainly to changes in:
   A. Blood pressure
   B. Hormones
   C. Oxygen levels

7. Which holds the primary functions of respiratory regulation and circulation control by responding to changes in arterial partial pressure of oxygen (pO_2), partial pressure of carbon dioxide (pCO_2), and acid-base balance?
   A. Baroreceptors
   B. Chemoreceptors
   C. Placenta

8. In the neonate, a normally formed umbilical cord contains:
   A. One artery, two veins
   B. One vein, two arteries
   C. Two veins, two arteries

9. Most drugs cross the placenta via which mechanism?
   A. Active transport
   B. Facilitated diffusion
   C. Passive diffusion

10. Which of the following describes the function of the umbilical vein?
    A. Carries carbon dioxide from the fetus back to the placenta
    B. Carries deoxygenated blood from the fetus to the placenta
    C. Carries oxygenated blood from the placenta to the fetus

11. The fetus responds to a significant drop in partial pressure of oxygen (pO_2) by:
    A. Increasing oxygen consumption
    B. Reducing lactic acid production
    C. Shifting blood to vital organs

(See answers next page.)

1. A) Decrease
Maturation of the fetal vagus nerve leads to a decrease in the baseline FHR.

2. B) Heart rate (HR)
Fetal compensation for decreased maternal circulating volume occurs by increasing the fetal HR. CO increases in response to changes in HR or SV ($CO = HR \times SV$). The fetal heart operates near its peak; SV does not change significantly. Therefore, the only way to increase the CO is to increase the fetal HR. While increased fetal movement may increase the fetal HR, it is the increase in HR, not the fetal movement, that provides compensation.

3. B) Sinoatrial (SA) node
The FHR is controlled by the SA node. The AV node coordinates the electrical signal between the atria and the ventricles. The sympathetic nervous system plays a major role in the successful transition from fetal to neonatal life. While it may increase the heart rate (HR), the sympathetic nervous system does not regulate the HR.

4. B) Ductus venosus
The ductus venosus connects the umbilical vena cava, allowing well-oxygenated blood to enter the fetal heart and bypass the liver. The ductus arteriosus carries medium-oxygenated blood and serves to bypass the fetal lungs, protecting them from circulatory overload. The foramen ovale shunts highly oxygenated blood from the right to the left atrium.

5. B) Greater binding of oxygen
Compared to maternal blood, fetal blood has greater affinity for oxygen binding. It is easier for maternal blood to release oxygen into the tissues and stimulate erythropoietin release.

6. A) Blood pressure
Baroreceptors inform the autonomic nervous system of beat-to-beat changes in blood pressure within the arterial system, especially considering their location in the carotid sinuses and aortic arch. Chemoreceptors hold the primary functions of respiratory regulation and circulatory control related to oxygen, carbon dioxide, and acid-base balance.

7. B) Chemoreceptors
Chemoreceptors hold the primary functions of respiratory regulation and circulatory control related to oxygen, carbon dioxide, and acid-base balance. Baroreceptors inform the autonomic nervous system of beat-to-beat changes in blood pressure within the arterial system, especially considering their location in the carotid sinuses and aortic arch. The placenta serves as the conduit between the pregnant patient and the fetus for the exchange of oxygen, carbon dioxide, and nutrients. It does not regulate fetal respiratory or circulatory functions.

8. B) One vein, two arteries
A normally formed umbilical cord contains one vein and two arteries. An abnormal umbilical cord may contain one vein and one artery and is referred to as a single umbilical artery.

9. C) Passive diffusion
Most drugs cross the placenta via passive or simple diffusion as it does not require energy or a carrier. Drugs that require transport via facilitated diffusion do not require energy but do require a carrier, whereas drugs that cross via active transport require energy.

10. C) Carries oxygenated blood from the placenta to the fetus
The function of the umbilical vein is to carry oxygenated blood from the placenta to the fetus. The umbilical arteries carry deoxygenated blood, including carbon dioxide, from the fetus to the placenta.

11. C) Shifting blood to vital organs
Just like an adult, the fetus responds to a significant drop in oxygen supply by shifting blood to vital organs. Increasing oxygen consumption and reducing lactic acid production do not occur in the fetus when oxygen supplies are low.

12. Which of the following is associated with the following fetal tracing?

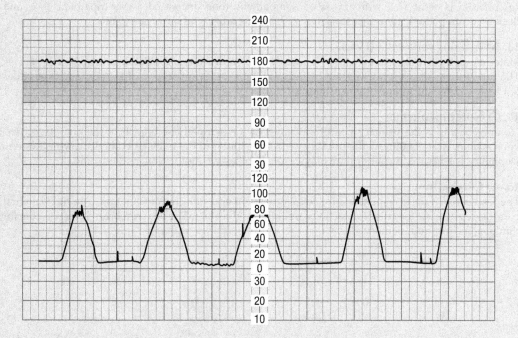

 A. Decreased sympathetic tone
 B. Increased parasympathetic tone
 C. Increased sympathetic tone

13. Maternal supine hypotension is caused primarily by compression of the:
 A. Inferior vena cava (IVC)
 B. Superior vena cava
 C. Uterine vessels

14. Which of the following is the primary neurotransmitter of the sympathetic branch of the autonomic nervous system?
 A. Acetylcholine
 B. Dopamine
 C. Norepinephrine

15. Which of the following is responsible for fetal muscle coordination?
 A. Cerebellum
 B. Cerebral cortex
 C. Cerebrum

(*See answers next page.*)

12. C) Increased sympathetic tone

Tachycardia is associated with increased sympathetic tone. Increased parasympathetic tone and decreased sympathetic tone are associated with a decreasing fetal heart rate (FHR).

13. A) Inferior vena cava (IVC)

Maternal supine hypotension is caused primarily by compression of the IVC due to the gravid uterus. The superior vena cava is not affected by the gravid uterus. Compression of the uterine vessels does not lead to maternal supine hypotension.

14. C) Norepinephrine

Norepinephrine is the primary neurotransmitter of the sympathetic branch of the autonomic nervous system. Acetylcholine is the primary neurotransmitter of the parasympathetic nervous system. Dopamine is a neurotransmitter than plays a role in pleasure, motivation, and learning.

15. A) Cerebellum

The fetal cerebellum is responsible for fetal movement and muscle coordination. The fetal cerebral cortex is responsible for voluntary actions, thinking, and feeling. The fetal cerebrum is responsible for thinking, feeling, and memory.

▶ REFERENCES

Abuhamad, A. Z., Shaffer, W., Mari, G., Copel, J. A., Hobbins, J. C., & Evans, A. T. (1995). Single umbilical artery: Does it matter which artery is missing? *American Journal of Obstetrics and Gynecology, 173*(3 Pt 1), 728–732. https://doi.org/10.1016/0002-9378(95)90331-3

Audus, K. L. (1999). Controlling drug delivery across the placenta. *European Journal of Pharmaceutical Sciences, 8*(3), 161–165.

Barrios-Arpi, L. M., Rodríguez Gutiérrez, J. L., & Lopez-Torres, B. (2017). Histological characterization of umbilical cord in alpaca (Vicugna pacos). *Anatomia, Histologia, Embryologia, 46*(6), 533–538. https://doi.org/10.1111/ahe.12298

Beall, M. H., van den Wijngaard, J. P., van Gemert, M. J., & Ross, M. G. (2007). Amniotic fluid water dynamics. *Placenta, 28*(8–9), 816–823. https://doi.org/10.1016/j.placenta.2006.11.009

Blazer, S., Sujov, P., Escholi, Z., Itai, B. H., & Bronshtein, M. (1997). Single umbilical artery—Right or left? Does it matter? *Prenatal Diagnosis, 17*(1), 5–8. https://doi.org/10.1002/(sici)1097-0223(199701)17:1<5::aid-pd999>3.0.co;2-4

Budorick, N. E., Kelly, T. F., Dunn, J. A., & Scioscia, A. L. (2001). The single umbilical artery in a high-risk patient population: What should be offered? *Journal of Ultrasound in Medicine, 20*(6), 619–628. https://doi.org/10.7863/jum.2001.20.6.619

Campbell, J., Wathen, N., Macintosh, M., Cass, P., Chard, T., & Mainwaring Burton, R. (1992). Biochemical composition of amniotic fluid and extraembryonic coelomic fluid in the first trimester of pregnancy. *British Journal of Obstetrics and Gynaecology, 99*(7), 563–565. https://doi.org/10.1111/j.1471-0528.1992.tb13821.x

Creasy, R., Resnik, R., Iams, J., Lockwood, C., Moore, T., & Greene, M. (2019). *Creasy & Resnik's maternal-fetal medicine: Principles and practice* (8th ed.). Elsevier.

Desforges, M., & Sibley, C. P. (2009). Placental nutrient supply and fetal growth. *International Journal of Developmental Biology, 54*(2–3), 377–390.

Eshkoli, T., Sheiner, E., Ben-Zvi, Z., Feinstein, V., & Holcberg, G. (2011). Drug transport across the placenta. *Current Pharmaceutical Biotechnology, 12*(5), 707–714.

Feliks, M., & Howorka, E. (1968). Znaczenie czynnościowe wezłów rzekomych pepowiny [functional value of false knots of the umbilical cord]. *Ginekologia Polska, 39*(6), 617–624.

Finnemore, A., & Groves, A. (2015). Physiology of the fetal and transitional circulation. *Seminars in Fetal & Neonatal Medicine, 20*(4), 210–216. https://doi.org/10.1016/j.siny.2015.04.003

Freeman, R., Garite, T., Nageotte, M., & Miller, L. (2012). *Fetal heart rate monitoring* (4th ed.). Wolters Kluwer.

Geipel, A., Germer, U., Welp, T., Schwinger, E., & Gembruch, U. (2000). Prenatal diagnosis of single umbilical artery: Determination of the absent side, associated anomalies, Doppler findings and perinatal outcome. *Ultrasound in Obstetrics & Gynecology, 15*(2), 114–117. https://doi.org/10.1046/j.1469-0705.2000.00055.x

Griffiths, S., & Campbell, J. (2015). Placental structure, function and drug transfer. *Continuing Education in Anaesthesia Critical Care & Pain, 15*(2), 84–89.

Gude, N. M., Roberts, C. T., Kalionis, B., & King, R. G. (2004). Growth and function of the normal human placenta. *Thrombosis Research, 114*(5–6), 397–407. https://doi.org/10.1016/j.thromres.2004.06.038

Hooper, S. B., Polglase, G. R., & te Pas, A. B. (2015). A physiological approach to the timing of umbilical cord clamping at birth. *Archives of Disease in Childhood: Fetal and Neonatal Edition, 100*(4), F355–F360. https://doi.org/10.1136/archdischild-2013-305703

Kehl, S., Schelkle, A., Thomas, A., Puhl, A., Meqdad, K., Tuschy, B., Berlit, S., Weiss, C., Bayer, C., Heimrich, J., Dammer, U., Raabe, E., Winkler, M., Faschingbauer, F., Beckmann, M. W., & Sütterlin, M. (2016). Single deepest vertical pocket or amniotic fluid index as evaluation test for predicting adverse pregnancy outcome (SAFE trial): A multicenter, open-label, randomized controlled trial. *Ultrasound in Obstetrics & Gynecology, 47*(6), 674–679. https://doi.org/10.1002/uog.14924

Kim, J. H., Jin, Z. W., Murakami, G., Chai, O. H., & Rodríguez-Vázquez, J. F. (2018). Persistent right umbilical vein: A study using serial sections of human embryos and fetuses. *Anatomy & Cell Biology, 51*(3), 218–222. https://doi.org/10.5115/acb.2018.51.3.218

King, T., & Parer, J. (2000). The physiology of fetal heart rate patterns and perinatal asphyxia. *Journal of Perinatal and Neonatal Nursing, 14*(3), 19–38. https://doi.org/10.1097/00005237-200012000-00003

Knipp, G. T., Audus, K. L., & Soares, M. J. (1999). Nutrient transport across the placenta. *Advanced Drug Delivery Reviews, 38*(1), 41–58.

Kornacki, J., Adamczyk, M., Wirstlein, P., Osiński, M., & Wender-Ożegowska, E. (2017). Polyhydramnios—Frequency of congenital anomalies in relation to the value of the amniotic fluid index. *Ginekologia Polska, 88*(8), 442–445. https://doi.org/10.5603/GP.a2017.0081.4

Lim, G., Facco, F. L., Nathan, N., Waters, J. H., Wong, C. A., & Eltzschig, H. K. (2018). A review of the impact of obstetric anesthesia on maternal and neonatal outcomes. *Anesthesiology, 129*(1), 192–215. https://doi.org/10.1097/ALN.0000000000002182

Lubusky, M., Dhaifalah, I., Prochazka, M., Hyjanek, J., Mickova, I., Vomackova, K., & Santavy, J. (2007). Single umbilical artery and its siding in the second trimester of pregnancy: Relation to chromosomal defects. *Prenatal Diagnosis, 27*(4), 327–331. https://doi.org/10.1002/pd.1672

Mamatha, H., Hemalatha, B., Vinodini, P., Souza, A. S. D., & Suhani, S. (2015). Anatomical study on the variations in the branching pattern of internal iliac artery. *Indian Journal of Surgery, 77,* 248–252.

Menihan, C., & Kopel-Puretz, E. (2019). *Electronic fetal monitoring—Concepts and applications* (3rd ed.). Wolters Kluwer.

Miller, L., Miller, D., & Cypher, R. (2017). *Fetal monitoring: A multidisciplinary approach* (8th ed.). Mosby Elsevier.

Moore, T. R. (2011). The role of amniotic fluid assessment in evaluating fetal well-being. *Clinics in Perinatology, 38*(1), 33–46. https://doi.org/10.1016/j.clp.2010.12.005

Morton, S. U., & Brodsky, D. (2016). Fetal physiology and the transition to extrauterine life. *Clinics in Perinatology, 43*(3), 395–407. https://doi.org/10.1016/j.clp.2016.04.001

Mushambi, M. (2002). Physiology of pregnancy. In C. Pinnock, T. Lin, & T. Smith (Eds.), *Fundamentals of Anaesthesia,* (pp. 484–498). Cambridge University Press. https://doi.org/10.1017/CBO9780511641947.028.

Olaya-C, M., & Bernal, J. E. (2015). Clinical associations to abnormal umbilical cord length in Latin American newborns. *Journal of Neonatal-Perinatal Medicine, 8*(3), 251–256. https://doi.org/10.3233/NPM-15915056

Pacifici, G. M., & Nottoli, R. (1995). Placental transfer of drugs administered to the mother. *Clinical Pharmacokinetics, 28,* 235–269.

Painter, D., & Russell, P. (1977). Four-vessel umbilical cord associated with multiple congenital anomalies. *Obstetrics and Gynecology, 50*(4), 505–507.

Sepulveda, W., Shennan, A. H., Bower, S., Nicolaidis, P., & Fisk, N. M. (1995). True knot of the umbilical cord: A difficult prenatal ultrasonographic diagnosis. *Ultrasound in Obstetrics & Gynecology, 5*(2), 106–108. https://doi.org/10.1046/j.1469-0705.1995.05020106.x

Shevell, T., Malone, F. D., Vidaver, J., Porter, T. F., Luthy, D. A., Comstock, C. H., Hankins, G. D., Eddleman, K., Dolan, S., Dugoff, L., Craigo, S., Timor, I. E., Carr, S. R., Wolfe, H. M., Bianchi, D. W., D'Alton, M. E., & FASTER Research Consortium. (2005). Assisted reproductive technology and pregnancy outcome. *Obstetrics & Gynecology, 106*(5 Part 1), 1039–1045.

Suliburska, J., Kocyłowski, R., Komorowicz, I., Grzesiak, M., Bogdański, P., & Barałkiewicz, D. (2016). Concentrations of mineral in amniotic fluid and their relations to selected maternal and fetal parameters. *Biological Trace Element Research, 172*(1), 37–45. https://doi.org/10.1007/s12011-015-0557-3

Suwanrath, C., & Suntharasaj, T. (2010). Sleep–wake cycles in normal fetuses. *Archives of Gynecology and Obstetrics, 281*(3), 449–454. https://doi.org/10.1007/s00404-009-1111-3

Tong, X. L., Wang, L., Gao, T. B., Qin, Y. G., Qi, Y. Q., & Xu, Y. P. (2009). Potential function of amniotic fluid in fetal development—Novel insights by comparing the composition of human amniotic fluid with umbilical cord and maternal serum at mid and late gestation. *Journal Chinese Medical Association, 72*(7), 368–373. https://doi.org/10.1016/S1726-4901(09)70389-2

Ullberg, U., Lingman, G., Ekman-Ordeberg, G., & Sandstedt, B. (2001). Hyrtl's anastomosis is normally developed in placentas from small for gestational age infants. *Acta Obstetricia et Gynecologica Scandinavica, 82*(8), 716–721. https://doi.org/10.1034/j.1600-0412.2003.00161.x

Yanaihara, A., Hatakeyama, S., Ohgi, S., Motomura, K., Taniguchi, R., Hirano, A., Takenaka, S., & Yanaihara, T. (2018). Difference in the size of the placenta and umbilical cord between women with natural pregnancy and those with IVF pregnancy. *Journal of Assisted Reproduction and Genetics, 35*(3), 431–434. https://doi.org/10.1007/s10815-017-1084-2

Assessment of Fetal Oxygenation and Acid-Base Status

Shannon Riley DaSilva

▶ INTRODUCTION

Fetal hypoxia is a major contributor to stillbirth, hypoxic ischemic encephalopathy (HIE), and cerebral palsy. Intrapartum-related fetal hypoxia is a common cause of neonatal encephalopathy, which includes a decreased level of consciousness or seizures, respiratory dysfunction, altered tone, altered reflexes, cerebral palsy, intellectual impairment, deafness, and blindness (American Academy of Pediatrics, 2014). Intrapartum-related hypoxia-ischemia is one of the top three causes of neonatal death globally (GBD 2019 Under-5 Mortality Collaborators, 2021). The opportunity to intervene quickly in cases of fetal hypoxia to prevent hypoxic injury or fetal death is the rationale for the use of electronic fetal heart rate (FHR) monitoring.

▶ OBJECTIVES

- Understand the physiology of fetal oxygenation.
- Understand respiratory, mixed, and metabolic acidemia.
- Analyze cord blood gas results.
- Identify neonatal signs consistent with an acute peripartum or intrapartum ischemic-hypoxic event.
- Understand information reflected in the umbilical artery and umbilical vein cord gases.
- Identify disruptions in the oxygenation pathway for the fetus.
- Identify electronic fetal monitoring (EFM) FHR patterns suggesting fetal acid-base balance.
- Identify FHR patterns suggesting fetal hypoxia.

▶ KEY TERMS

- **Acidemia:** Decreased pH of the blood caused by an increase in hydrogen ion concentration
- **Acidosis:** Increased hydrogen ions in tissue or decreased pH in tissue
- **Asphyxia:** Hypoxia with metabolic acidosis
- **Hypoxia:** Decreased oxygen content in the tissues
- **Hypoxemia:** Decreased oxygen content in the blood
- **Metabolic acidosis:** Pathologic process that increases the concentration of hydrogen ions (H^+) and reduces blood bicarbonate (HCO_3) concentration
- **Mixed acidemia:** Low pH with elevated partial pressure of carbon dioxide (pCO_2) and base deficit (BD)
- **Respiratory acidosis:** Elevation in arterial partial pressure of carbon dioxide ($PaCO_2$) concentration that reduces arterial pH and normal HCO_3 levels

▶ PHYSIOLOGY OF FETAL OXYGENATION

Maternal physiologic changes occur during pregnancy to support the adequate oxygenation of the fetus. The placenta acts as the fetal lungs and is responsible for fetal acid-base balance and respiratory blood gas homeostasis.

MATERNAL PHYSIOLOGIC CHANGES AND FETAL ACID-BASE BALANCE

The pregnancy state is associated with a reduction in maternal pCO_2. This change is thought to facilitate diffusion of blood gases between the fetal and the maternal circulations. With adequate buffering, the maternal arterial pH has minimal change. The maternal state is one of compensated respiratory alkalosis and enhanced renal secretion of acid. Circulatory changes, an increased potential for oxygen-hemoglobin dissociation, and maternal hyperventilation help to facilitate oxygen transfer across the placenta and maintain maternal acid-base balance in pregnancy. The fetus produces acids in normal metabolism and maintains extracellular pH with an efficient buffer system, primarily by the production of plasma HCO_3 and hemoglobin. Very small changes in pH can have a significant impact on the functions of fetal organ systems, including the central nervous system and the cardiovascular system (Omo-Aghoja, 2014).

▶ PRINCIPLES OF ACID-BASE PHYSIOLOGY

Fetal oxygenation requires transfer of oxygen from the pregnant patient to the fetus and an adequate fetal response. The oxygen is transferred from the maternal lungs, heart, vasculature, uterus, and placenta to the umbilical cord, then to the fetus. This oxygen transfer can be interrupted at any point and at multiple points. Different pathologic processes can disrupt the oxygen flow as it passes through each system (Figure 4.1).

PATHOLOGIC CONDITIONS' IMPACT ON THE OXYGENATION PATHWAY

Adequate oxygenation of the maternal lungs is disrupted by pathologic conditions such as asthma, apnea during seizures, medications, and pneumonia. Maternal anemia and hemoglobinopathies can decrease the oxygen-carrying capacity in the maternal vasculature. Vasoconstriction from chronic hypertension, diabetes, and renal disease also affects the maternal vasculature. Preeclampsia is known to cause vascular remodeling at the spiral arteries of the placenta, impacting its perfusion. Regional anesthesia can cause maternal hypotension and interrupt fetal oxygenation.

FETAL RESPONSE

Once the oxygen is transferred to the fetus through the placenta, the fetal hemoglobin has a higher affinity for oxygen, resulting in increased oxygen-carrying capacity. Fetal anemia, fetal-maternal hemorrhage, and fetal hemoglobinopathies can reduce the fetal ability to adequately oxygenate. Certain complications in pregnancy, such as oligohydramnios, can cause umbilical cord compression and thus disrupt oxygenated blood adequately reaching the fetus.

LABOR PROCESS AND FETAL OXYGENATION

The labor process contributes to fetal acid-base changes. The latent phase of labor results in minimal change in fetal umbilical artery BD (Ross, 2021). During the active phase, the BD increases approximately 1 mmol/L every 3 to 6 hours, and in the second stage, it increases approximately 1 mmol/L per hour of active pushing (Ross, 2021). Contractions during normal labor interrupt the oxygen transfer by impacting the uterus. Normal labor contractions create a short period of hypoxia that a healthy fetus compensates for to maintain an acid-base balance. The fetus in most cases is shielded by the normal hypoxic effects of the labor process with an adequate placenta function and sufficient maternal oxygen perfusion. The fetus responds through a compensatory process with disruptions in the oxygen pathway. Initially, in periods of reduced blood flow or decreased oxygen, the fetus shunts the blood from the inactive muscle groups to protect the brain, heart, and adrenals (Turner et al., 2020). Excessive uterine activity can interrupt the oxygen transfer to the fetus. Studies have shown that the presence of excessive uterine activity without the appearance of FHR changes can result in fetal acidemia (Bakker et al., 2007; Caldeyro-Barcia, 1992). Ongoing hypoxia and acidosis reduce the myocardial glycogen stores (needed for aerobic and anaerobic metabolism), impair cardiac function, and cause systemic hypotension and ultimately multiorgan damage (Turner et al., 2020).

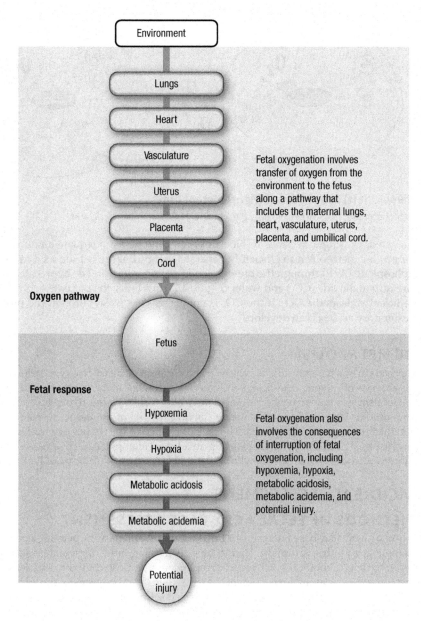

Figure 4.1 Physiology of the Fetal Oxygen Pathway.

Clinical Pearl

Normal labor contractions create a short period of hypoxia that a healthy fetus compensates for to maintain acid-base balance.

▶ FETAL METABOLISM OF ENERGY

AEROBIC METABOLISM

Maternal oxygenation, adequate placental function, and sufficient umbilical cord perfusion are necessary for fetal oxygenation in an uncompromised fetus. Hypoxemia occurs when the fetus is

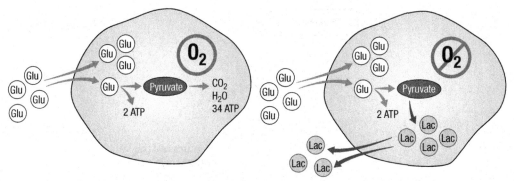

Figure 4.2 Aerobic (left) and anaerobic (right) metabolism.

ATP, adenosine triphosphate; CO_2, carbon dioxide; glu, glucose; H_2O, water; lac, lactic acid.

not well oxygenated, causing a decrease in blood oxygen content. An adequate amount of oxygen is required for aerobic metabolism to efficiently generate energy. Energy is produced in the form of adenosine triphosphate (ATP) through the breakdown of glycogen stores. The byproducts of aerobic metabolism are carbon dioxide (CO_2) and water (Figure 4.2). In a fetus, the placenta acts as lungs and quickly and efficiently clears the CO_2. If the CO_2 is not excreted as waste through the placenta in a timely way, respiratory acidosis can develop.

ANEROBIC METABOLISM

Continued deprivation of oxygen results in hypoxia. Hypoxia is a decrease in oxygenation of the fetal tissues. In the absence of oxygen, the tissues convert to anaerobic metabolism to generate energy. Anaerobic metabolism generates energy less efficiently and results in the byproduct of lactic acid. Buffer bases are used as lactic acid accumulates to stabilize the pH of the tissues. Metabolic acidosis develops when the buffer system is depleted. The lack of oxygen in the tissues eventually progresses to acidemia and asphyxia. Metabolic acidosis results in a lower fetal pH. An Apgar score of less than 5 at 5 or 10 minutes correlates with a low newborn blood pH (American Academy of Pediatrics, 2014).

▶ FETAL ACID-BASE ASSESSMENT

DIRECT METHODS OF FETAL ACID-BASE ASSESSMENT

Direct evaluation of fetal acid-base balance can be assessed by antepartum percutaneous umbilical cord blood sampling, by intrapartum fetal scalp blood sampling, and immediately after birth by umbilical cord sampling. Umbilical cord blood sampling is the most common and least invasive method for assessing the fetal acid-base balance. While there is no consensus on when to collect umbilical cord acid-base analysis, it is commonly collected with a low Apgar score at 5 minutes, a category III FHR pattern, or following an operative vaginal delivery. In cases of maternal, fetal, or obstetric problems with known risk of neonatal depression, a clinician may consider preemptively collecting a cord segment. This allows the healthcare team to wait and collect gases from the segment until the status of the newborn is known.

Collecting Blood Gases With Delayed Cord Clamping

Delaying the collection on the umbilical cord may affect pH and gas values due to continuing metabolism and diffusion of the gases. Collecting a specimen after delaying cord clamping for up to 2 minutes has been shown to have little or no effect on the results (Nudelman et al., 2020). Safe and accurate cord blood gas samples can be obtained from an unclamped pulsating umbilical artery and vein if cord clamping is delayed (Xodo et al., 2018).

INTERPRETATION OF CORD BLOOD GASES

The pH, pCO_2, partial pressure of oxygen (pO_2), hemoglobin, and oxygen content of the blood are measured. The pH and BD are the most useful values when interpreting the fetal acid-base status. The reference range for umbilical artery blood gas values in a preterm newborn is shown in Chapter 2, Table 2.5, and the reference range for umbilical artery blood gas values in a term newborn is shown in Chapter 2, Table 2.4. A pH of less than 7 is defined as the pathologic fetal acidemia threshold (American Academy of Pediatrics, 2014). There are three types of acidosis: mixed, metabolic, and respiratory acidemia. Respiratory acidemia results in a low pH and a high pCO_2 with a normal HCO_3 concentration. Mixed acidemia includes a low pH, a low HCO_3 concentration, and a high pCO_2. Metabolic acidemia includes a low pH, a normal pCO_2, and a low HCO_3 concentration. A metabolic component is associated with increased risk of neonatal morbidity and mortality (Andres et al., 1999). The BD is calculated from pH and pCO_2.

Clinical Pearl

A metabolic component is associated with increased risk of neonatal morbidity and mortality.

BASE DEFICIT FROM EXTRACELLULAR FLUID

Recent reports emphasize that BD from extracellular fluid (ECF) should be used instead of BD from blood values. The ECF value is interpreted by the lab using the blood obtained from the umbilical artery. BD of ECF gives a clearer picture than BD of blood due to the elevated levels of pCO_2 that commonly occurs in fetal umbilical artery blood samples, especially with end-labor bradycardia (Ross, 2021). BD of blood values are significantly increased when compared with BD of ECF due to the elevated pCO_2 levels (Ross, 2021).

ASSESSING UMBILICAL VEIN BLOOD GASES

Most clinicians collect both umbilical artery and umbilical vein samples. Collecting both allows the samples to be compared. Umbilical venous values can also be informative in determining the timing of a hypoxic event. Umbilical artery blood is preferred because it reflects fetal metabolism, whereas the umbilical vein blood reflects placental function. In situations where the flow from the fetus to the placenta is stopped, such as with umbilical cord occlusion or complete placental separation, the values obtained from the umbilical vein represent the fetal values at the time of the event (Ross, 2021). The umbilical artery levels represent the newborn status at the time of birth, which could be remote from a sentinel event. With such an event, fetal umbilical artery pCO_2 initially increases by approximately 7 mmHg per minute due to the absent CO_2 clearance by the placenta (Ross, 2021). Umbilical vein levels offer information regarding the placental state prior to the acute event and allow evaluation on the timing of the occurrence of cord occlusion or placental separation (Ross, 2021).

Clinical Pearl

Umbilical artery blood reflects fetal metabolism, while umbilical vein blood reflects placental function.

▶ ELECTRONIC FETAL MONITORING

EFM initially was intended to reduce the incidence of neurologic injury, such as cerebral palsy, caused by fetal hypoxia. However, routine use of EFM has not been shown to decrease events of cerebral palsy as expected. Evidence suggests that approximately 70% of cerebral palsy cases occur prior to labor onset and are unrelated to intrapartum events (American College of Obstetrics and Gynecology [ACOG], 2009).

LIMITATIONS OF ELECTRONIC FETAL MONITORING

The efficacy of EFM has been scrutinized for its ability to decrease complications without causing unnecessary interventions. EFM has been shown to increase the overall Cesarean rate and increase operative vaginal deliveries (ACOG, 2009). EFM has not been shown to reduce perinatal mortality or the risk of cerebral palsy and has a false-positive rate of greater than 99% for predicting cerebral palsy. EFM has a poor interobserver and intraobserver reliability and an uncertain efficacy (ACOG, 2009).

The literature consistently supports a normal fetal acid-base status with the presence of moderate variability and/or accelerations (ACOG, 2009). In other words, if an FHR pattern shows moderate variability and/or accelerations, the healthcare team can be reassured that the fetus is adequately oxygenated at the time of the observation. The FHR pattern is limited to the fetal status at the time of observation. It does not allow the healthcare team to know if a prior event has already caused injury to the fetus. A study by Clark et al. (2018) suggests that under ideal circumstances only half of infants born with fetal metabolic acidemia could have been potentially identified with EFM and had an expedited delivery.

Clinical Pearl

FHR tracings with the presence of moderate variability and/or accelerations reflect a normal fetal acid-base status.

CONSENSUS OF CAUSAL LINKS BETWEEN INTRAPARTUM HYPOXIC EVENTS AND NEONATAL NEUROLOGIC INJURY

The American College of Obstetrics and Gynecology (ACOG) Task Force on Neonatal Encephalopathy formed a widely accepted consensus regarding causal links between intrapartum hypoxic events and cerebral palsy (American Academy of Pediatrics, 2014). Based on the consensus, neonatal signs that are consistent with an acute event, either intrapartum or peripartum, include an Apgar score less than 5 at 5 minutes and 10 minutes, fetal umbilical artery acidemia, specific findings on neonatal brain imaging, presence of neonatal multisystem organ failure, presence of a sentinel event before delivery, and FHR patterns consistent with an acute event.

Fetal Umbilical Artery Acidemia and Development of Cerebral Palsy

Significant fetal umbilical artery acidemia is defined as a pH less than 7.0 or a BD greater than or equal to 12 mmol/L or both (American Academy of Pediatrics, 2014). Additional studies show that a BD greater than or equal to 20 mmol/L further increases the incidence of cerebral palsy (Ross, 2021). The rate of cerebral palsy with a BD of 12 to 19.9 mmol/L ranges from 2.1% to 4% and increases to 33% with a BD of 20 mmol/L (Ross, 2021). Most infants with acidemia at birth do not develop cerebral palsy. Additionally, to prevent the development of cerebral palsy, an obstetric intervention must be done prior to the BD reaching 12 mmol/L (Ross, 2021).

Neonatal Hypoxic Neurologic Injury and Fetal Brain Imaging

Accurate interpretation and expertise in neonatal neuroradiology are necessary to determine if a neurologic injury occurred from an acute peripartum or intrapartum event. Specific types of brain injury patterns on imaging are consistent with an etiology of an acute peripartum or intrapartum hypoxic-ischemic event. The timing and type of imaging to evaluate fetal brain injury are important in interpretation.

Fetal Brain Imaging Modalities

Ultrasonography lacks sensitivity; however, it is sometimes the only option for a very unstable infant (American Academy of Pediatrics, 2014). Echodensity and echogenicity on ultrasonography can be detected for 48 hours or longer after an ischemic cerebral injury (American Academy of Pediatrics, 2014). A CT lacks sensitivity and may not reveal an abnormality in the 24 to 48 hours after injury (American Academy of Pediatrics, 2014). MRI and magnetic resonance spectroscopy are the most sensitive modalities to evaluate the timing of cerebral injury.

MRI Use for Assessment of Neonatal Neurologic Injury

An MRI is the most common and most useful modality to identify if the ischemic event was an acute peripartum or intrapartum event. MRI performed between 24 and 96 hours of life can provide useful information regarding the timing of an insult. Diffusion abnormalities are most prominent between 24 and 96 hours and are most evident after 7 days (American Academy of Pediatrics, 2014). Evaluation at day 10 of life or later assists in evaluating the extent of the cerebral injury (American Academy of Pediatrics, 2014). Patterns of brain injury that are typical of hypoxic-ischemic cerebral injury include deep nuclear gray matter or watershed cortical injury (American Academy of Pediatrics, 2014).

Clinical Pearl

An MRI is the most common and most useful modality to identify if an ischemic event was an acute peripartum or intrapartum event.

Fetal Acidemia Following a Sentinel Event

Fetal acidemia noted after a sentinel event such as uterine rupture, severe abruptio placentae, umbilical cord prolapse, amniotic fluid embolism, maternal cardiac collapse, or fetal-maternal hemorrhage meets criteria as inclusion in a causal link for an intrapartum hypoxic event. This casual relationship is due to the clear disruption of the oxygenation pathway to the fetus. A sentinel event that results in an acute fetal hypoxic event likely will also have associated abnormal FHR patterns.

Fetal Heart Rate Patterns and Fetal Acid-Base Status

A three-tier categorization of the FHR tracing is used and reflects the predicted fetal acid-base status. Category I FHR tracings predict a normal fetal acid-base status. The literature consistently supports that the presence of moderate variability and/or accelerations correlates with a normal fetal acid-base balance (ACOG, 2009). Persistent category III tracings are abnormal and are associated with a risk for abnormal fetal acid-base status at the time of observation. Category III tracings require prompt evaluation and intervention. When assessing an FHR pattern, it is important to consider the underlying fetal acid-base status. Absent or minimal variability is caused by blunting of the parasympathetic outflow that reduces the moment-to-moment regulation of the FHR due to metabolic acidemia. Variable decelerations, recurrent late decelerations, and bradycardia, as discussed earlier in the chapter, are associated with fetal acidemia. It is important to interpret the EFM pattern in context and consider additional factors that can influence the findings. For example, fetal sleep cycles, medications, and prematurity are other potential causes for decreased FHR variability.

Clinical Pearl

Persistent category III tracings are associated with possible abnormal fetal-acid base status at the time visualized.

Category II Fetal Heart Rate Pattern

A category II tracing is indeterminate and requires continued surveillance and reevaluation. The management of a category II FHR pattern offers many challenges when monitoring the FHR. According to the consensus on neonatal ischemic injury, a category II tracing lasting 60 minutes or longer, identified on initial presentation with persistent minimal or absent variability and lacking accelerations even in the absence of decelerations, suggests a previously compromised fetus (American Academy of Pediatrics, 2014). Certain changes in FHR tracings have been shown in the literature to be consistent with an acute intrapartum event. For example, a neonate born with acidemia is likely the result of an acute intrapartum event if the patient presented with a category I tracing and converted to a category III tracing (American Academy of Pediatrics, 2014). Additionally, an acute intrapartum event is also likely if a previous category I tracing developed tachycardia with recurrent decelerations or progressed to persistent minimal variability with recurrent decelerations (American Academy of Pediatrics, 2014).

The literature suggests using ancillary tests to aid in the management of a category II pattern. These tests include fetal scalp sampling, Allis clamp scalp stimulation, vibroacoustic stimulation, and digital scalp stimulation. Most often, the less invasive vibroacoustic or digital stimulation is used and preferred. When an acceleration follows stimulation, acidemia is unlikely (ACOG, 2009). Early decelerations are not associated with increase in the fetal umbilical artery BD (Ross, 2021). Variable decelerations and late decelerations may increase the BD (Ross et al., 2013). Fetal bradycardia between 50 and 70 bpm increases the BD by 1 mmol/L for every 2 minutes (Hagelin & Leyon, 1998). In animal models, a BD can be cleared at a rate of approximately .1 mmol/L per minute (Ross et al., 2013). The impact of the labor process, disruptions in the pathway of fetal oxygenation, and disruptions in the fetal clearance of acid are all factors contributing to the fetal acid-base balance.

Clinical Pearl

When an acceleration follows vibroacoustic or digital scalp stimulation, fetal acidemia is unlikely.

Approaches for Management of a Category II Fetal Heart Rate Pattern

Continued research and approaches have been developed to offer further clarity in management of a category II FHR pattern. In 2013, an algorithm was published with recommendations for management of category II tracings (Clark et al., 2013). The algorithm assists the clinician in deciding if continued observation versus expedited delivery is necessary based on the presence of persistent significant decelerations for a period with or without moderate variability or accelerations. The guidelines of the algorithm were established based on the ACOG consensus criteria regarding hypoxic-ischemic events and EFM patterns. The foundational principle of managing the category II tracing according to the algorithm includes considering the likelihood of significant acidemia developing prior to delivery (Clark et al., 2013). The article suggests that applying the algorithm "along with the integration of future evidence-based modifications driven by additional research, will provide clinicians with a standardized, simple, rational, evidence-based, and nationally accepted approach to the management of Category II FHR patterns" (Clark et al., 2013).

Fetal Reserve Indicators

Emerging research is focusing on fetal reserve indicators (FRIs). EFM alone is narrowly focused and ignores contextual issues such as maternal, fetal, and obstetric risk factors (Evans et al., 2022). The FRI approach contextualizes the EFM interpretation with increased uterine activity and various maternal, obstetric, and fetal risk factors. The risk factors are categorized based on their effect on the oxygenation pathways and fetal response. Fetal reserve index scoring could offer clarity on the risk of fetal metabolic acidemia. For example, a category II tracing in the presence of fetal meconium would alert at a higher risk level than without fetal meconium (Pruksanusak et al., 2022). Implementing this approach may be helpful in correctly identifying fetal acidemia and allow appropriate intervention.

Fetal Heart Rate Patterns and Underlying Fetal Acid-Base Status

It is important to understand the underlying fetal response and fetal acid-base status when interpreting FHR patterns. An early deceleration is described as a symmetrical decrease and return of FHR that is associated with a uterine contraction. The decrease in an early deceleration is gradual, with the onset to the nadir 30 seconds or longer, and mirrors the contraction. Multiple animal studies conclude that this response is related to head compression eliciting a response due to reduced cerebral blood flow and intracranial pressure (Fodstad et al., 2006). Late, variable, and prolonged decelerations are caused by an interruption of oxygen pathways. Late decelerations are a response to temporary oxygen interruption during a contraction (American Academy of Pediatrics, 2014). A late deceleration can be a physiologic response or a pathologic response to the oxygen pathway disruption. Physiologically, the fetal blood oxygen decrease triggers chemoreceptors to cause reflex constriction of blood vessels in nonvital peripheral areas to divert more blood flow to vital organs such as the adrenal glands, heart, and brain. The constriction of peripheral blood vessels results in hypertension. The hypertension stimulates a baroreceptor-mediated vagal response and slows the heart rate (HR). The time taken is a delay from the insult of hypoxia caused by the contraction, which explains why the deceleration nadir is after the peak of the contraction (Harris et al., 1982). Late decelerations have a pathologic etiology due to marked fetal acidemia leading to myocardial depression (Martin, 2008).

Variable decelerations result from mechanical umbilical cord compression. A prolonged deceleration also represents a disruption in oxygen to the fetus and can be caused by maternal hemodynamic changes, cord compression, uteroplacental perfusion, and excessive uterine activity. Characteristics of decelerations are discussed in Chapter 6.

Clinical Pearl

Late, variable, and prolonged decelerations are caused by an interruption of the oxygen pathway from the patient to the fetus.

Management of Abnormal Fetal Heart Rate Patterns

Management approaches have been developed to aid the clinician in intervening appropriately after an abnormal FHR pattern is recognized to attempt to remedy the insult disrupting fetal oxygenation. One approach of management is the A, B, C, D method (Miller & Miller, 2012). The clinician (A) assesses the oxygen pathway, (B) begins corrective measures, (C) clears obstacles to rapid delivery, and (D) develops a delivery plan (Miller & Miller, 2012). A disruption in fetal oxygenation can occur along any of the pathways of oxygenation to the fetus from the maternal lungs, maternal heart, maternal vasculature, uterus, and placenta to the umbilical cord. Assessing the cause of the oxygenation disruption and beginning the appropriate corrective measure are the first two steps in the A, B, C, D approach. For example, a variable deceleration is noted on the FHR tracing. Variable decelerations are due to cord compression, implementing the corrective measures of maternal position change, reduced uterine activity, and possibly initiating an amnioinfusion. Clearing obstacles for delivery includes addressing any source of delay of delivery, including those from facility, staff, patient, fetus, and labor. They can include completion of consent forms and laboratory tests, availability of specialists such as anesthesia providers, and operating room availability.

▶ KEY POINTS

- Hypoxia is a major contributor to neonatal morbidity and mortality.
- The opportunity to intervene quickly in cases of fetal hypoxia and prevent hypoxic injury or fetal death is the rationale for the use of EFM.
- Maternal physiologic changes occur during pregnancy to support the fetus.
- The placenta acts as the fetal lungs and is responsible for fetal acid-base balance and respiratory blood gas homeostasis.
- The fetus responds to disruptions in the oxygenation pathways through compensatory processes.
- Decreased fetal oxygenation and fetal hypoxia can be reflected in FHR patterns.
- Moderate variability and/or accelerations reflect an oxygenated fetus.
- Persistent category III tracings reflex hypoxemia of the fetus.

CASE STUDY

Addison is a 31-year-old G2P1001 patient presenting to labor and delivery at 40 weeks and 2 days' gestation. She reports spontaneous contractions beginning approximately 5 hours ago. The cervical exam is 7/100/-2. Initial vital signs are blood pressure (BP) 132/86 mmHg, HR 76, respiratory rate (RR) 16, and oxygen saturation (SpO$_2$) 99%. She is requesting an epidural for pain management. After 1 hour of a category I tracing, an epidural is placed, and the patient is put supine with a left tilt following the procedure. Her vital signs are now BP 92/62 mmHg, HR 112, RR 16, and SpO$_2$ 98%. Late decelerations are noted with minimal variability. The bedside nurse repositions the patient to left lateral and administers an IV bolus. The patient's BP returns to baseline of 130/82 mmHg. Spontaneous rupture of membranes reveals thin meconium. Throughout the remaining 5 hours of labor, the fetus demonstrates intermittent variable and late decelerations with periods of both minimal and moderate variability. During the patient's 1-hour second stage, a 3-minute prolonged deceleration to the 60s with absent variability occurs 5 minutes before delivery. Addison delivers a live male infant weighing 8 lb 6 oz with Apgar scores of 2, 5, and 7 at 1, 5, and 10 minutes, respectively. Examination of the placenta reveals a placental abruption. The infant responds to positive pressure ventilation and is transferred to the NICU. Arterial cord blood gases are collected, revealing pH 6.75, pCO$_2$ 51, pO$_2$ 18, and BD 18.5. The infant is diagnosed with neonatal encephalopathy.

Answer the following, and then see the Case Study Answers for correct answers.

1. What does interpretation of the arterial cord blood gases reveal?

2. What conclusion can be drawn about the status of the fetus?

3. The bedside nurse's actions after the epidural focused on which disruption in the oxygenation pathway for the fetus: maternal lungs, maternal heart, maternal vasculature, or uterus?

(See answers next page.)

CASE STUDY ANSWERS

1. Metabolic acidemia. pH is less than 7, pCO_2 is within normal range, and BD is above 12.

2. The FHR tracing suggests an acute hypoxic-ischemic event during the intrapartum period. A neonate born with acidemia is likely the result of an acute intrapartum event if the patient presents with a category I tracing that converts to a category III tracing.

3. Maternal vasculature. Hypotensive BP following the epidural disrupted the fetal oxygenation. An IV fluid bolus can improve fetal oxygenation by increasing maternal cardiac output, venous return, left ventricular preload, and stroke volume.

KNOWLEDGE CHECK: CHAPTER 4

1. The most common cause of cerebral palsy is:
   A. A complication resulting from a congenital anomaly
   B. An acute peripartum or intrapartum hypoxic-ischemic event
   C. An event that occurred prior to labor onset

2. What may be concluded from review of the fetal heart rate (FHR) pattern noted in the following?

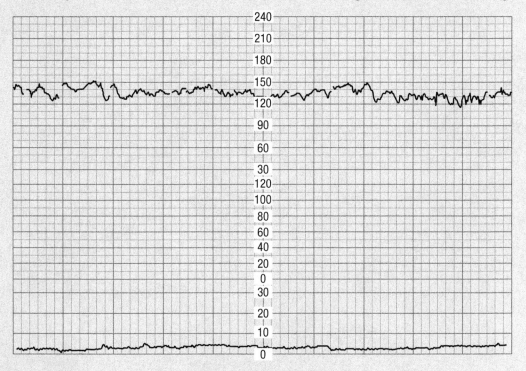

   A. Category I tracing with signs of fetal oxygenation as evidenced by moderate variability
   B. Category II tracing with signs of fetal hypoxia as evidenced by absent accelerations
   C. Category II tracing with signs of fetal oxygenation as evidenced by moderate variability

(See answers next page.)

1. C) An event that occurred prior to labor onset

Evidence suggests that approximately 70% of cerebral palsy cases occur prior to labor onset and are unrelated to intrapartum events. Most infants with acidemia at birth do not develop cerebral palsy. Most causes of cerebral palsy are not the result of a congenital anomaly.

2. A) Category I tracing with signs of fetal oxygenation as evidenced by moderate variability

The literature consistently supports a normal fetal acid-base status with the presence of moderate variability and/or accelerations. The tracing is category I, not category II.

3. The bedside nurse notes the fetal heart rate (FHR) pattern shown in the following and demonstrates understanding of the pathway of disruption for fetal oxygenation by implementing which intervention?

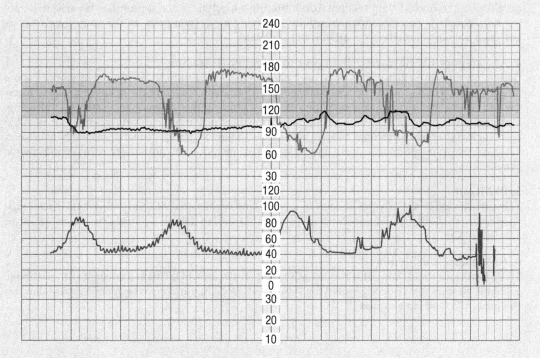

A. Administering a tocolytic to the patient
B. Applying an oxygen mask to the patient
C. Recommending an amnioinfusion to the provider

4. A patient presents to labor and delivery in active labor. Prenatal care was uncomplicated with no significant medical or surgical history. The initial electronic fetal monitoring (EFM) fetal heart rate (FHR) tracing is category I with an FHR baseline of 150, moderate variability, and accelerations noted. The FHR tracing changes to a category II tracing with minimal to moderate variability. Thirty minutes before birth, the FHR tracing is a category III tracing with absent variability and recurrent variable decelerations. The neonate is born 8 hours after admission with umbilical artery pH of 6.59 and Apgar scores of 1, 5, and 7 at 1 minute, 5 minutes, and 10 minutes, respectively. The neonate is transferred to the NICU for cooling after resuscitation and intubation and is diagnosed with neonatal encephalopathy. What findings are consistent with an intrapartum hypoxic-ischemic event?
A. Category I FHR tracing changing to category III tracing
B. Diagnosis of neonatal encephalopathy
C. Uncomplicated prenatal care with no significant medical or surgical history

5. The clinician is evaluating the results of umbilical artery blood gas testing: pH 6.89, pressure of carbon dioxide (pCO_2) 96, base deficit (BD) 20. These results are consistent with which kind of acidemia?
A. Metabolic
B. Mixed
C. Respiratory

6. The clinician is evaluating the results of umbilical artery blood gases: pH 6.89, pressure of carbon dioxide (pCO_2) 49, base deficit (BD) 13. These results indicate:
A. Metabolic acidemia
B. Mixed acidemia
C. Respiratory acidemia

(See answers next page.)

3. C) Recommending an amnioinfusion to the provider

The nurse correctly identifies variable decelerations, which are related to umbilical cord compression leading to disruption of fetal oxygenation. An amnioinfusion has been shown to resolve variable decelerations from cord compression. Administering a tocolytic is not appropriate because this tracing does not show excessive uterine activity. Applying an oxygen mask to the pregnant patient is indicated only if maternal oxygenation is not adequate.

4. A) Category I FHR tracing changing to category III tracing

Certain changes in FHR tracings have been shown in the literature to be consistent with an acute intrapartum event. For example, a neonate born with acidemia is likely the result of an acute intrapartum event if the patient presents with a category I tracing that converts to a category III tracing. Uncomplicated prenatal care with no significant medical or surgical history can rule out possible pathologic causes of the outcome, but it is not associated with an intrapartum hypoxic-ischemic event. Neonatal encephalopathy can have multiple causes, including an intrapartum hypoxic-ischemic event.

5. B) Mixed

These results indicate a low pH, an elevated pCO_2, and an elevated BD, indicating mixed acidemia. Respiratory acidemia would not show an elevated BD, and metabolic acidemia would not show an elevated pCO_2.

6. A) Metabolic acidemia

These results indicate a low pH, a normal pCO_2, and an elevated BD. This is consistent with metabolic acidemia. Respiratory acidemia would not show an elevated BD, and mixed acidemia would show an elevated pCO_2 with an elevated BD.

7. A 38-year-old G2P1001 patient at 38 weeks and 1 day's gestation is admitted to the ICU with complications from pneumonia secondary to influenza A. oxygen saturation (SpO_2) is 85% and is slowly increased to 98% with the application of a nonrebreather oxygen mask. The nurse notes a category III tracing after initiating electronic fetal monitoring (EFM). The neonate is delivered by emergency Cesarean with umbilical artery blood gases showing pH 6.75, pressure of carbon dioxide (pCO_2) 129, and base deficit (BD) 19. The likely oxygen disruption pathway that led to this outcome is the maternal:
   A. Heart
   B. Lungs
   C. Vasculature

8. A 41-year-old G5P3012 patient at 38 weeks and 3 days' gestation presents to labor and delivery. The initial electronic fetal monitoring (EFM) tracing is category II with minimal variability and recurrent late decelerations. The umbilical artery cord gases show metabolic acidemia, and the neonate is transferred after resuscitation and intubation to the NICU. The maternal complications of pregnancy included chronic hypertension with superimposed preeclampsia, preexisting diabetes managed by insulin, and advanced maternal age. Which of the following caused the oxygenation pathway disruption and increased the risk of fetal acidemia?
   A. Preeclampsia and vasoconstriction from chronic hypertension and diabetes are both causes of oxygen pathway disruption
   B. Preeclampsia is known to cause vascular remodeling at the spiral arteries of the placenta, impacting the placental oxygenation pathway to the fetus
   C. Vasoconstriction from chronic hypertension and diabetes impacts fetal oxygenation due to disruptions in maternal vasculature

9. The clinician notes an acceleration of the fetal heart rate (FHR) following digital fetal scalp stimulation. Which of the following is supported by current evidence and the literature?
   A. The healthcare team decides to continue labor because acidemia is unlikely with an acceleration following fetal scalp stimulation
   B. The healthcare team expedites delivery by Cesarean section due to the association between fetal acidemia and acceleration after fetal scalp stimulation
   C. The healthcare team takes no action because fetal scalp stimulation has not been shown to give evidence-based information on fetal pH status

10. Umbilical artery cord gases may be delayed up to how many minutes without having an effect on the results?
   A. 1
   B. 2
   C. 3

11. Pathologic fetal acidemia is defined as an umbilical cord artery pH of less than:
   A. 6.5
   B. 7.0
   C. 7.5

12. Intrapartum-related hypoxia is one of the top three causes of neonatal death globally and is the most common cause of:
   A. Neonatal encephalopathy
   B. Neonatal necrotizing enterocolitis
   C. Retinopathy of prematurity

(See answers next page.)

7. B) Lungs
The oxygenation of the maternal lungs was disrupted by the patient's pneumonia. The maternal heart and maternal vasculature were not disrupted.

8. A) Preeclampsia and vasoconstriction from chronic hypertension and diabetes are both causes of oxygen pathway disruption
Vasoconstriction from chronic hypertension, diabetes, and renal disease affects the maternal vasculature. Preeclampsia is known to cause vascular remodeling at the spiral arteries of the placenta, impacting its perfusion.

9. A) The healthcare team decides to continue labor because acidemia is unlikely with an acceleration following fetal scalp stimulation
Digital scalp stimulation is a less invasive procedure than fetal scalp sampling to aid in assessing fetal pH. When there is an acceleration following scalp stimulation, acidemia is unlikely. The healthcare team may decide to continue labor. An acceleration following fetal scalp stimulation is not associated with fetal acidemia. Fetal scalp stimulation is used in clinical practice to aid in assessing fetal pH.

10. B) 2
Delaying collection on the umbilical cord may affect pH and the gas values due to continuing metabolism and diffusion of the gases. A specimen collected after delaying cord clamping for up to 2 minutes has been shown to have little or no effect on the results. Safe and accurate cord blood gas samples can be obtained from an unclamped pulsating umbilical artery and vein if cord clamping is delayed.

11. B) 7.0
A pH of less than 7 is defined as the pathologic fetal acidemia threshold.

12. A) Neonatal encephalopathy
Fetal hypoxia is a major contributor to stillbirth, HIE, and cerebral palsy. Intrapartum-related fetal hypoxia is a common cause of neonatal encephalopathy, which includes a decreased level of consciousness or seizures, respiratory dysfunction, altered tone, altered reflexes, cerebral palsy, intellectual impairment, deafness, and blindness. Intrapartum-related hypoxia-ischemia is one of the top three causes of neonatal death globally. Neonatal necrotizing enterocolitis and retinopathy of prematurity are not directly caused by fetal hypoxia.

13. Which of the following is *true* concerning the following fetal heart rate (FHR) tracing?

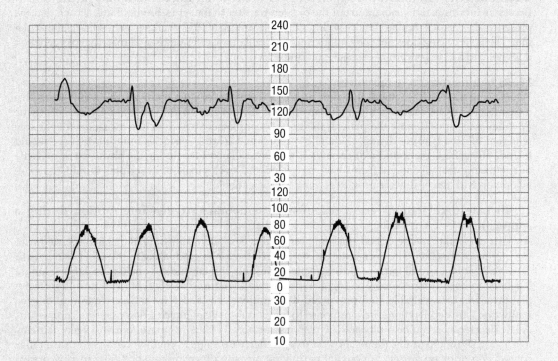

A. The FHR pattern shows signs of likely fetal oxygenation with the presence of moderate variability and accelerations

B. The healthcare team should apply oxygen to the pregnant patient to increase maternal oxygen and increase fetal oxygenation

C. The healthcare team should attempt to decrease uterine activity because excessive uterine activity can interrupt oxygen transfer to the fetus and result in fetal acidemia

14. The nurse notices maternal hypotension after epidural placement. The fetal heart rate (FHR) tracing shows late decelerations with moderate variability. The nurse increases the IV fluids and repositions the patient to the left lateral position. Increasing the IV fluids and repositioning the patient are evidence of the nurse's application of which step in the ABCD management method?

A. Begins corrective measures

B. Clears obstacles to rapid delivery

C. Develops a delivery plan

15. Which of the following statements correctly describes the etiology of a deceleration?

A. Early decelerations are caused by the response of the fetus to hypoxic events with normal labor contractions

B. Late decelerations are a response to temporary oxygen interruption during a contraction

C. Variable decelerations are due to marked fetal acidemia leading to myocardial depression

(See answers next page.)

13. C) The healthcare team should attempt to decrease uterine activity because excessive uterine activity can interrupt oxygen transfer to the fetus and result in fetal acidemia
Excessive uterine activity can interrupt the oxygen transfer to the fetus. Studies have shown that the presence of excessive uterine activity without the appearance of FHR changes can result in fetal acidemia. The FHR tracing does not show moderate variability or accelerations, and maternal oxygenation does not correct the concern of excessive uterine activity.

14. A) Begins corrective measures
When using the ABCD method, the clinician (A) assesses the oxygen pathway, (B) begins corrective measures, (C) clears obstacles to rapid delivery, and (D) develops a delivery plan. By increasing the IV fluids and repositioning the patient, the nurse is implementing corrective measures for the low maternal BP that is likely disrupting fetal oxygenation. Clearing obstacles to rapid delivery would include any actions that could reduce barriers to delivery, such as notifying the physician or midwife or confirming that all consent forms have been signed. Developing a delivery plan would be in collaboration with the healthcare provider caring for the patient.

15. B) Late decelerations are a response to temporary oxygen interruption during a contraction
An early deceleration is described as a symmetrical decrease and return of FHR that is associated with the uterine contraction. The decrease in an early deceleration is gradual, with the onset to the nadir 30 seconds or longer, and mirrors the contraction. Multiple animal studies conclude that this response is related to head compression eliciting a response due to reduced cerebral blood flow and intracranial pressure. Late, variable, and prolonged decelerations are caused by an interruption of oxygen pathways. Late decelerations are a response to temporary oxygen interruption during a contraction. A late deceleration can be a physiologic response or a pathologic response to the oxygen pathway disruption. Physiologically, the fetal blood oxygen decrease triggers chemoreceptors to cause reflex constriction of blood vessels in nonvital peripheral areas to divert more blood flow to vital organs such as the adrenal glands, heart, and brain. The constriction of peripheral blood vessels results in hypertension. The hypertension stimulates a baroreceptor-mediated vagal response and slows the HR. The time taken is a delay from the insult of hypoxia caused by the contraction, which explains why the deceleration nadir is after the peak of the contraction. Late decelerations have a pathologic etiology due to marked fetal acidemia leading to myocardial depression. Variable decelerations result from mechanical umbilical cord compression.

▶ REFERENCES

American Academy of Pediatrics. (2014). Neonatal encephalopathy and neurologic outcome, second edition. *Pediatrics*, *133*(5), e1482–e1488. https://doi.org/10.1542/peds.2014-0724

American College of Obstetrics and Gynecology. (2009). ACOG practice bulletin 106. Intrapartum fetal heart rate monitoring: Nomenclature, interpretation, and general management principles. *Obstetrics and Gynecology*, *114*(1), 192–202. https://doi.org/10.1097/AOG.0b013e3181aef106

Andres, R. L., Saade, G., Gilstrap, L. C., Wilkins, I., Witlin, A., Zlatnik, F., & Hankins, G. V. (1999). Association between umbilical blood gas parameters and neonatal morbidity and death in neonates with pathologic fetal acidemia. *American Journal of Obstetrics and Gynecology*, *181*(4), 867–871. https://doi.org/10.1016/s0002-9378(99)70316-9

Bakker, P., Kurver, P., Kuik, D., & Van Geijn, H. (2007). Elevated uterine activity increases the risk of fetal acidosis at birth. *American Journal of Obstetrics Gynecology*, *196*(4), 313 e1–313 e6. https://doi.org/10.1016/j.ajog.2006.11.035

Caldeyro-Barcia, R. (1992). Intrauterine fetal reanimation in acute intrapartum fetal distress. *Early Human Development*, *29*(1–3), 27–33. https://doi.org/10.1016/0378-3782(92)90054-k

Clark, S. L., Garite, T. J., Hamilton, E. F., Belfort, M. A., & Hankins, G. D. (2018). "Doing something" about the cesarean delivery rate. *American Journal of Obstetrics Gynecology*, *219*(3), 267–271. https://doi.org/10.1016/j.ajog.2018.04.044

Clark, S. L., Nageotte, M. P., Garite, T. J., Freeman, R. K., Miller, D. A., Simpson, K. R., Belfort, M. A., Dildy, G. A., Parer, J. T., Berkowitz, R. L., D'Alton, M., Rouse, D. J., Gilstrap, L. C., Vintzileos, A. M., van Dorsten, J. P., Boehm, F. H., Miller, L. A., & Hankins, G. D. (2013). Intrapartum management of Category II fetal heart rate tracings: Towards standardization of care. *American Journal of Obstetrics Gynecology*, *209*(2), 89–97. https://doi.org/10.1016/j.ajog.2013.04.030

Evans, M. I., Britt, D. W., Evans, S. M., & Devoe, L. D. (2022). Changing perspectives of electronic fetal monitoring. *Reproductive Sciences*, *29*(6), 1874–1894. https://doi.org/10.1007/s43032-021-00749-2

Fodstad, H., Kelly, P. J., & Buchfelder, M. (2006). History of the cushing reflex. *Neurosurgery*, *59*(5), 1132–1137. https://doi.org/10.1227/01.NEU.0000245582.08532.7C

GBD 2019 Under-5 Mortality Collaborators. (2021). Global, regional, and national progress towards sustainable development goal 3.2 for neonatal and child health: All-cause and cause-specific mortality findings from the global burden of disease study 2019. *The Lancet*, *398*(10303), 870–905. https://doi.org/10.1016/S0140-6736(21)01207-1

Hagelin, A., & Leyon, J. (1998). The effect of labor on the acid-base status of the newborn. *Acta Obstetricia Et Gynecologica Scandinavica*, *77*(8), 841–844.

Harris, J. L., Krueger, T. R., & Parer, J. T. (1982). Mechanisms of late decelerations of the fetal heart rate during hypoxia. *American Journal of Obstetrics and Gynecology*, *144*(5), 491–496. https://doi.org/10.1016/0002-9378(82)90215-0

Martin, C. B. Jr. (2008). Normal fetal physiology and behavior, and adaptive responses with hypoxemia. *Seminars in Perinatology*, *32*(4), 239–242. https://doi.org/10.1053/j.semperi.2008.04.003

Miller, D. A., & Miller, L. A. (2012). Electronic fetal heart rate monitoring: Applying principles of patient safety. *American Journal of Obstetrics and Gynecology*, *206*(4), 278–283. https://doi.org/10.1016/j.ajog.2011.08.016

Nudelman, M., Belogolovsky, E., Jegatheesan, P., Govindaswami, B., & Song, D. (2020). Effect of delayed cord clamping on umbilical blood gas values in term newborns: A systematic review. *Obstetrics & Gynecology*, *135*(3), 576–582. https://doi.org/10.1097/AOG.0000000000003663

Omo-Aghoja, L. (2014). Maternal and fetal acid-base chemistry: A major determinant of perinatal outcome. *Annals of Medical and Health Sciences Research*, *4*(1), 8–17. https://doi.org/10.4103/2141-9248.126602

Pruksanusak, N., Chainarong, N., Boripan, S., & Geater, A. (2022). Comparison of the predictive ability for perinatal acidemia in neonates between the NICHD 3-tier FHR system combined with clinical risk factors and the fetal reserve index. *PLoS One*, *17*(10), e0276451. https://doi.org/10.1371/journal.pone.0276451

Ross, M. (2021). Forensic analysis of umbilical and newborn blood gas values for infants at risk of cerebral palsy. *Journal of Clinical Medicine*, *10*(8), 1676. https://doi.org/10.3390/jcm10081676

Ross, M., Jessie, M., Amaya, K., Matushewski, B., Durosier, L., Frasch, M., & Richardson, B. S. (2013). Correlation of arterial fetal base deficit and lactate changes with severity of variable heart rate decelerations in the near-term ovine fetus. *American Journal of Obstetrics and Gynecology, 208*, e281–e286. https://doi.org/10.1016/j.ajog.2012.10.883

Turner, J., Mitchell, M., & Kumar, S. (2020). The physiology of intrapartum fetal compromise at term. *American Journal of Obstetrics and Gynecology, 222*(1), 17–26. https://doi.org/10.1016/j.ajog.2019.07.032

Xodo, S., Xodo, L., & Berghella, V. (2018). Delayed cord clamping and cord gas analysis at birth. *Acta Obstetricia Et Gynecologica Scandinavica, 97*(1), 7–12. https://doi.org/10.1111/aogs.13233

Maternal, Fetal, and Placental Complications

Shannon Riley DaSilva

▶ INTRODUCTION

Maternal, fetal, and placental complications in pregnancy include a wide range of conditions that have minor to major implications and risks to the pregnant patient and fetus. This chapter is a brief overview of the more common complications encountered in pregnancy. Most of the complications covered in this chapter have some degree of impact on uteroplacental function.

Antepartum fetal surveillance is often indicated to assess fetal status. Different techniques for surveillance include cardiotocography (electronic fetal monitoring, or EFM) and ultrasonography. The goal of such surveillance is to identify suspected fetal compromise and intervene before metabolic acidosis progresses to fetal death. Some acute events, such as with intrahepatic cholestasis or a severe placental abruption, may not be identified in a timely way with EFM or ultrasound surveillance. Commonly performed antepartum fetal tests for surveillance are the nonstress test, biophysical profile, fetal growth assessment, middle cerebral artery velocimetry, and umbilical artery Doppler velocimetry (American College of Obstetricians and Gynecologists [ACOG], 2021a). The type of test performed, the frequency of the test, and the gestational age at which antepartum fetal testing starts depend on the severity of the condition and the fetal risks associated with the condition (ACOG, 2021a).

▶ OBJECTIVES

- ▪ Review common maternal complications of pregnancy.
- ▪ Understand maternal and fetal risks with common maternal complications of pregnancy.
- ▪ Review common placental complications of pregnancy.
- ▪ Understand maternal and fetal risks with common placental complications of pregnancy.
- ▪ Review common fetal complications of pregnancy.
- ▪ Understand maternal and fetal risks with common fetal complications of pregnancy.
- ▪ Identify, if indicated, the impact of pregnancy complications on fetal heart rate (FHR) patterns.

▶ KEY TERMS

- ▪ **Antepartum fetal surveillance/antepartum fetal tests:** Techniques used to assess the fetal status, typically through EFM or ultrasonography
- ▪ **Coagulopathy:** Any condition affecting the blood's ability to clot
- ▪ **Hypoxemia:** Decreased oxygen content in blood
- ▪ **Hypoxia:** Decreased oxygen content in tissues
- ▪ **Idiopathic:** Of unknown cause
- ▪ **Ischemia:** Inadequate blood supply to an organ or part of the body
- ▪ **Metabolic acidosis:** Pathologic process that increases the concentration of hydrogen ions (H^+) and reduces blood bicarbonate (HCO_3) concentration
- ▪ **Thrombocytopenia:** Low platelets ($<150 \times 10^9/L$)

▶ MATERNAL COMPLICATIONS

HYPERTENSIVE DISORDERS OF PREGNANCY

Hypertensive disorders of pregnancy (HDPs) include both chronic and pregnancy-associated hypertension. HDPs are responsible for 14% of maternal deaths worldwide and almost 8% of maternal deaths in the United States (Say et al., 2014). The incidence of HDPs increased from 13.3% to 15.9% from 2017 to 2019 among delivery hospitalizations (Ford et al., 2022).

Preeclampsia

The incidence of preeclampsia has also increased. This is likely related to the population increase in risk factors for preeclampsia. Risk factors for preeclampsia include multifetal gestations, preeclampsia in a previous pregnancy, chronic hypertension, pregestational diabetes, gestational diabetes, thrombophilia, autoimmune disease (systemic lupus erythematosus [SLE], antiphospholipid antibody syndrome), pre-pregnancy body mass index (BMI) greater than 30, maternal age 35 years or older, kidney disease, nulliparity, family history of preeclampsia in first-degree relative, use of assisted reproductive technology, and obstructive sleep apnea (Louis et al., 2022).

Preeclampsia is caused by underlying abnormal placentation resulting in placental dysfunction. While the mechanism of abnormal placentation is controversial, evidence shows that genetic, maternal/environmental, and immunologic factors lead to abnormal placentation. Abnormal placentation causes oxidative stress, persistent hypoxia, a proinflammatory state, and maternal endothelial dysfunction, ultimately leading to systemic vascular dysfunction (Rana et al., 2019). Systemic vascular dysfunction manifests as proteinuria from glomerular endotheliosis; hypertension; cerebral edema/visual disturbances/headaches, seizures (eclampsia); and coagulation abnormalities/hemolysis, elevated liver enzymes, and a low platelet (HELLP) syndrome.

Preeclampsia prevention research is ongoing. Multiple studies show a reduction in preeclampsia and fetal growth restriction with low-dose aspirin when started between 12 and 28 weeks' gestation. Therefore, the ACOG and the Society for Maternal-Fetal Medicine (SMFM) recommend the use of low-dose aspirin in people at high risk for preeclampsia or with multiple moderate risk factors. Diagnostic criteria for gestational hypertension include systolic blood pressure ≥140 mmHg or diastolic blood pressure ≥90 mmHg on two occasions 4 hours apart after 20 weeks' gestation with previously normal blood pressure. A preeclampsia diagnosis is made when a patient who meets criteria for gestational hypertension also has proteinuria (greater than 300 mg per 24-hour urine collection, protein creatinine ratio of .3 or more, or a dipstick reading of 2+ if no other quantitative methods are available; ACOG, 2020a). A diagnosis of preeclampsia can be made without proteinuria with gestational hypertension and new onset of one of the following: thrombocytopenia, renal insufficiency, impaired liver function, pulmonary edema, or new-onset headache unresponsive to medications and not accounted for by an alternative diagnosis or visual disturbances (ACOG, 2020a). A patient with severe-range blood pressures, systolic blood pressure ≥160 mmHg, or diastolic blood pressure ≥110 mmHg should be diagnosed with preeclampsia with severe features (ACOG, 2020a). Severe features include blood pressures in the severe-range levels, thrombocytopenia $<100 \times 10^9$/L, impaired liver function with liver enzymes more than twice the upper limit of normal or severe persistent right upper quadrant pain or epigastric pain, renal insufficiency with a serum creatinine more than 1.1 mg/dL or doubling, pulmonary edema, new-onset headache unresponsive to medications, or visual disturbances (ACOG, 2020a).

Clinical Pearl

Signs of preeclampsia with severe features include blood pressures in the severe-range levels, thrombocytopenia, impaired liver function, renal insufficiency, pulmonary edema, new-onset headache unresponsive to medications, or visual disturbances.

Maternal Risk

Patients with preeclampsia have hemoconcentration; they do not have the same increase in blood volume as in a normal pregnancy. Several vasodilators and vasoconstrictive agents interact, resulting in vasospasms (ACOG, 2020a). Those with preeclampsia have hyperdynamic ventricular function and low pulmonary capillary wedge pressure. The pulmonary capillary wedge pressure increases significantly with excessive IV fluids and puts the patient at risk for pulmonary edema. Hematologic changes may occur with preeclampsia with severe features and may reach severe levels as part of HELLP syndrome. Increased platelet activation, aggregation, and consumption in preeclampsia results in thrombocytopenia (a platelet count $<150 \times 10^9$/L). Lactate dehydrogenase (LDH) is elevated with hemolysis and hepatic dysfunction. Liver dysfunction can occur due to periportal and focal parenchymal necrosis, hepatic cell edema, and Glisson capsule distension. Serologic changes noted with elevated alanine aminotransferase (ALT) and aspartate aminotransferase (AST) reflect liver involvement. Renal changes cause increased tubular permeability of most large-molecular-weight proteins, causing proteinuria. The vasospasms lead to contraction of intravascular space and worsen renal sodium and water retention (ACOG, 2020a). Oliguria (<100 mL of urine output over 4 hours) can occur with severe preeclampsia due to the intrarenal vasospasms. Serum uric acid concentration may also increase in preeclampsia.

Maternal symptoms reflect the underlying pathophysiology of preeclampsia. Severe persistent right upper quadrant or epigastric pain unresolved with medications is due to liver involvement. New-onset headaches unresponsive to medications and visual disturbances are due to cerebral involvement. Maternal complications may also include myocardial infarction, pulmonary edema, stroke, acute respiratory distress syndrome, coagulopathy, renal failure, and retinal injury (ACOG, 2020a). Patients with a history of preeclampsia are at increased risk for cardiovascular disease (CVD) and dementia later in life (Rana et al., 2019). After experiencing preeclampsia, patients often have mental health sequelae such as posttraumatic stress disorder (PTSD) and anxiety (Louis et al., 2022).

Fetal Risk

Impaired uteroplacental blood flow resulting from the placental dysfunction limits blood flow to the uteroplacental unit, causing ischemia. Clinical manifestations from uteroplacental ischemia include fetal growth restriction, stillbirth, oligohydramnios (low amniotic fluid), placental abruption, and findings on antepartum surveillance that are suggestive of fetal hypoxia. Those with preeclampsia are at risk for spontaneous or medically indicated preterm delivery. Timing of delivery depends on the severity of the preeclampsia and the evaluation of the fetus. Expectant management allows fetal development until 37 weeks' gestation and is an option with gestational hypertension or preeclampsia without severe features. Expectant management includes serial monitoring of laboratory values, frequent antepartum fetal surveillance testing, daily home monitoring of maternal blood pressures, strict monitoring for signs of severe features, and weekly or twice weekly evaluation in a clinical setting of maternal symptoms and blood pressures (ACOG, 2020a). In the presence of severe features, eclampsia, HELLP, a fetus without expectation of survival, or abnormal fetal testing, expedited delivery is indicated.

Eclampsia

Eclampsia is a convulsive symptom of HDPs. It is characteristic of severe disease. The convulsions are new-onset, tonic-clonic, focal, or multifocal seizures in the absence of other causes such as epilepsy, cerebral arterial ischemia and infarction, drugs, or intracranial hemorrhages. Eclampsia can cause maternal death from severe hypoxia, trauma, and aspiration pneumonia (ACOG, 2020a). Long-term complications can include impaired memory and cognitive function. Maternal symptoms may occur prior to a seizure indicating signs of cerebral involvement. Symptoms include severe and persistent occipital or frontal headaches, blurred vision, photophobia, and altered mental status. Headaches are thought to be caused by cerebral edema, elevated perfusion pressure, and hypertensive encephalopathy (ACOG, 2020a). Eclampsia is not a necessarily a linear progression, from preeclampsia without severe features, to preeclampsia with severe features, to eclampsia. Studies have shown cases of eclampsia without any prior documentation of hypertension or proteinuria in a hospital setting (Xiao et al., 2022).

During an eclamptic seizure, the FHR pattern may show prolonged FHR decelerations or fetal bradycardia. Maternal hypoxia may cause recurrent decelerations, tachycardia, and reduced variability often seen after a seizure. Maternal stabilization often normalizes the fetal tracing, and delivery is recommended only after the patient is hemodynamically stabilized (ACOG, 2020a).

Clinical Pearl

FHR decelerations and sometimes fetal bradycardia can be seen during an eclamptic seizure. Recurrent decelerations, fetal tachycardia, and reduced variability may be noted after a seizure. FHR tracing often normalizes with maternal stabilization.

Hellp Syndrome

HELLP syndrome clinically presents as hemolysis, elevated liver enzymes, and a low platelet count. It is one of the more severe forms of preeclampsia and is associated with increased maternal morbidity and mortality. ACOG recommends using the following for the clinical criteria for diagnosis: LDH elevated to 600 IU/L or more, AST and ALT elevated to more than twice the upper limit of normal, and a platelet count less than 100×10^9/L (ACOG, 2020a). HELLP is most often seen in the third trimester but can also present postpartum. Patients may lack hypertension and proteinuria prior to the onset of HELLP syndrome. Most patients present with right upper quadrant pain, generalized malaise, and nausea and vomiting. Very close monitoring and expedited delivery are indicated in the presence of HELLP syndrome due to the high risk of adverse maternal and fetal outcomes. Adverse maternal outcomes include death, renal and hepatic failure, severe cardiac morbidity, disseminated intravascular coagulation (DIC), shock, obstetric embolism, sepsis, and eclampsia. Adverse fetal outcomes include perinatal death and severe morbidities such as intraventricular hemorrhage (Lisonkova et al., 2020).

TREATMENT OF HYPERTENSIVE DISORDERS OF PREGNANCY

Magnesium sulfate IV is given to prevent eclampsia in the presence of severe features with preeclampsia. Studies have shown that magnesium sulfate can reduce seizure rate, risk of placental abruption, and risk of maternal mortality (ACOG, 2020a). Magnesium sulfate is considered first-line for prevention of eclampsia, and it is also used in the presence of eclampsia to prevent recurrent convulsions. Alternatives may be considered if antiepileptic treatment is indicated or if magnesium sulfate is contraindicated or not available. Contraindications to magnesium sulfate include myasthenia gravis, hypocalcemia, moderate to severe renal failure, cardiac ischemia, heart block, pulmonary edema, or myocarditis (ACOG, 2020a). The most common side effect of magnesium sulfate is hot flashes. Adverse effects with magnesium toxicity include respiratory depression, pulmonary edema, cardiac arrest, and loss of deep tendon reflexes. Monitoring of urine output is important, as magnesium sulfate is excreted in the urine and the risk of oliguria is present with preeclampsia. Calcium gluconate 10% solution is used for emergency correction of magnesium toxicity.

Clinical Pearl

Magnesium sulfate is considered first-line for prevention of eclampsia, and it is also used in the presence of eclampsia to prevent recurrent convulsions.

Severe hypertension should be treated in a timely way with an antihypertensive agent to prevent congestive heart failure, myocardial ischemia, renal injury or failure, and ischemic or hemorrhagic stroke. With persistent (15 minutes or more), severe, acute-onset hypertension, antihypertensive agents should be administered within 30 to 60 minutes (ACOG, 2020a). Oral nifedipine, IV hydralazine, and IV labetalol are safe and effective medications to treat severe hypertension in pregnancy.

Chronic Hypertension

Chronic hypertension is defined as hypertension present before pregnancy or present before 20 weeks' gestation, or hypertension that persists beyond 12 weeks' postpartum (ACOG, 2019a). Diagnostic criteria from the American College of Cardiology (ACC) and the American Heart Association (AHA) describe four categories of blood pressure classification with accompanying recommendations (Table 5.1). ACOG defines hypertension in pregnancy as systolic blood pressure ≥140 mmHg and/or diastolic blood pressure ≥90 mmHg on two occasions at least 4 hours apart (ACOG, 2019a). SMFM recommends medication management for blood pressures that reach the threshold of 140/90 (SMFM, 2022). Severe hypertension in pregnancy is diagnosed as systolic blood pressure ≥160 mmHg or diastolic blood pressure ≥110 mmHg measured 4 hours apart; however, antihypertensive treatment should not be delayed. *White coat hypertension* is elevated blood pressure in the presence of healthcare providers. It is not benign and is associated with a risk of progression to gestational hypertension and preeclampsia.

Table 5.1 Blood Pressure Classification

Blood Pressure Category	Systolic Blood Pressure		Diastolic Blood Pressure
Normal	<120 mmHg	*and*	<80 mmHg
Elevated	120 to 129 mmHg	*and*	<80 mmHg
Hypertension			
Stage 1	130 to 139 mmHg	*or*	80 to 89 mmHg
Stage 2	≥140 mmHg	*or*	≥90 mmHg
Pregnancy			
Hypertension in prenatal period (two occasions 4 hours apart)	≥140 mmHg	*or*	≥90 mmHg
Severe-range hypertension (two occasions 4 hours apart)	≥160 mmHg	*or*	≥110 mmHg
Chronic Hypertension With or Without Preeclampsia			
Chronic hypertension without preeclampsia	Hypertension diagnosed or present before pregnancy or before 20 weeks' gestation; or hypertension that is diagnosed for the first time during pregnancy and that does not resolve in the postpartum period		
Chronic hypertension with superimposed preeclampsia	Preeclampsia in a patient with a history of hypertension before pregnancy or before 20 weeks' gestation		

Source: Data from Whelton, P., Carey, R., Aronow, W., Casey, D., Collins, K., Dennison Himmelfarb, C., DePalma, S., Gidding, S., Jamerson, K., Jones, D., MacLaughlin, E., Muntner, P., Ovbiagele, B., Smith, S., Spencer, C., Stafford, R., Taler, S., Thomas, R., Williams, K., Williamson, J., & Wright, J. (2018). 2017 ACC/AHA/AAPA/ABC/ACPM/AGS/APhA/ASH/ASPC/NMA/PCNA guidelines for the prevention, detection, evaluation, and management of high blood pressure in adults. *Hypertension*, *71*(19), e13–e115; American College of Obstetrics and Gynecology. (2019a). ACOG practice bulletin no. 203: Chronic hypertension in pregnancy. *Obstetrics and Gynecology, 133*(1), e26–e50. https://doi.org/10.1097/ AOG.0000000000003020.

Maternal Risks

Chronic hypertension increases the risk of maternal death, myocardial infarction, stroke, heart disease, pulmonary edema, renal failure, preeclampsia, and gestational diabetes and may indicate preterm birth (ACOG, 2019a). Compared to those without chronic hypertension, the risk of planned Cesarean delivery and postpartum hemorrhage is increased (ACOG, 2019a).

Fetal Risks

Chronic hypertension is associated with poor perinatal outcomes. Fetal risks include low birth weight, preterm delivery, fetal growth restriction, stillbirth, neonatal death, placenta abruption, and congenital anomalies (heart defects, hypospadias, esophageal atresia; ACOG, 2019a).

Chronic Hypertension: Electronic Fetal Monitoring Implications

The effect of chronic hypertension on FHR patterns is related to the underlying etiology. Fetal growth–restricted fetuses have fewer accelerations, higher risk of decelerations, and an increased rate of late decelerations (Cahill et al., 2013). Intrapartum use of antihypertensive medications given IV in term fetuses can result in decreased presence of accelerations (Graham et al., 2006). Data suggest that FHR changes cannot be reliably attributed to use of common oral antihypertensives but that underlying maternal or placental disease progression is likely a contributing factor to changes suggestive of fetal hypoxia (Waterman et al., 2004). Animal studies suggest that in the presence of a hypoxemic fetus, nifedipine can impair right ventricular function and reduce cardiac output, leading to FHR changes (Alanne et al., 2021). FHR responses to an eclamptic seizure include prolonged decelerations with fetal tachycardia after recovery from bradycardia (Ambia et al., 2022). Undetectable variability and bradycardia have been noted with severe placental abruption (Usui et al., 2008).

DIABETES IN PREGNANCY

Gestational Diabetes Mellitus

Gestational diabetes mellitus (GDM) is one of the most common complications of pregnancy. It is a condition of carbohydrate intolerance. Glucose uptake by the fetus and placenta causes fasting glucose levels to be lower in a normal pregnancy than in the nonpregnant state. Placental hormones cause mild postprandial elevated glucose levels and carbohydrate intolerance (American Diabetes Association [ADA], 2022). In normal pregnancies, the maternal pancreas can increase insulin production to compensate for elevated glucose levels. In gestational diabetes, the insulin response is inadequate (Egan et al., 2020). Distinguishing GDM from preexisting diabetes can be difficult due to a lack of diabetes screening prior to pregnancy. The prevalence of GDM is higher among Hispanic, African American, Native American, and Asian and Pacific Islander populations. Risk factors include obesity, increasing age, sedentary lifestyle, first-degree relatives with diabetes, hypertension, dyslipidemia, polycystic ovary syndrome (PCOS), CVD, HbA1C greater than or equal to 5.7%, impaired glucose tolerance or impaired fasting glucose, and prior GDM (ACOG, 2018a).

> ### Clinical Pearl
>
> Gestational diabetes is a condition of carbohydrate intolerance in pregnancy.

The U.S. Preventive Services Task Force (USPSTF) recommends screening all patients for GDM at 24 weeks' gestation or later (USPSTF et al., 2021). Early pregnancy screening for undiagnosed type 2 diabetes mellitus (DM) is suggested when the patient has risk factors for DM (ACOG, 2018a). Early testing should be performed at the initial visit. Screening for GDM is completed with a one-step or a two-step process. The one-step process is a test completed while fasting using a 75-g 2-hour oral glucose tolerance test (OGTT). Diagnosis is made if one of the three values is elevated. The two-step process includes completion of an initial 50-g 1-hour OGTT screen. The patient is not required to be fasting during the initial screening test. If the initial test is abnormal, the second step is a 100-g 3-hour diagnostic OGTT completed while fasting. If the initial 1-hour screening result is ≥200 mg/dL with a normal HbA1C, GDM is diagnosed without additional testing. The patient is diagnosed based on the two-step process if two of the four results are elevated. The HbA1C may also be used for early screening for preexisting diabetes but is not as sensitive when compared to OGTT (ADA, 2021). It is recommended to rescreen at 24 to 28 weeks even if the early screening is negative (ACOG, 2018a). Different thresholds are used for the OGTT results to diagnose GDM. Higher thresholds have a lower risk of false-positive rates and lower sensitivities. Lower thresholds have an increased risk of false-positive rates and risk of higher rates of GDM diagnosis in a lower-risk group. The one-step process has a higher rate of diagnosing GDM in those who may be at lower risk for adverse outcomes (ACOG, 2018a). The goal is appropriately testing and diagnosing GDM to treat effectively, leading to significant improvements in maternal and neonatal outcomes while also preserving healthcare costs and preventing unnecessary maternal stress and dissatisfaction.

Maternal and Fetal Risk

Patients with GDM are at increased risk for preeclampsia, Cesarean delivery, and developing diabetes later in life. Fetal risks include macrosomia, neonatal hypoglycemia, hyperbilirubinemia, polyhydramnios, shoulder dystocia, birth trauma, and stillbirth. Adequately controlling GDM reduces maternal and fetal risk factors. Diet changes focused on carbohydrate intake are the primary focus for glycemic control. Regular, consistent exercise is beneficial in controlling glucose levels. Frequent monitoring of blood sugars with a home glucometer, with assessment of fasting glucose levels and after meals helps determine glycemic control. The ADA and ACOG recommend fasting levels below 95 mg/dL and postprandial levels less than 140 mg/dL at 1 hour and 120 mg/dL at 2 hours (ADA, 2022). Increased antepartum fetal surveillance and serial fetal growth monitoring are recommended to assess for complications related to uncontrolled diabetes such as macrosomia, polyhydramnios, and frequent fetal assessment due to risk of stillbirth. Pharmacologic treatment is indicated when target glucose levels are not achieved with diet and exercise. Insulin is recommended as first line due to its ability to achieve tight glucose control and its safety profile as it does not cross the placenta (ACOG, 2018a). Oral antidiabetic medications are used when the patient declines insulin, it cannot be administered safely, or the patient cannot afford it. Oral antidiabetic medications cross the placenta, and there is concern about long-term neonatal effects after in utero exposure. Carbohydrate intolerance with GDM frequently resolves after delivery; however, screening for diabetes at 4 to 12 weeks postpartum is recommended. Some patients may have had undiagnosed preexisting diabetes, and between 15% and 70% of those who had GDM will develop diabetes later in life (ACOG, 2018a).

Pregestational Diabetes Mellitus

Pregestational DM is a challenging complication of pregnancy that requires frequent monitoring and medication adjustments and includes significant risk for the patient and fetus. Type 1 pregestational DM is caused by an autoimmune process that destroys the pancreatic beta cells, requiring insulin therapy. Type 1 DM is frequently seen earlier in life and has increased risk of development of vascular, renal, and neuropathic complications. Type 2 DM is due to peripheral insulin resistance and insulin deficiency and is more common later in life. The prevalence of pregestational DM is increased in patients of color, particularly African American, Native American, and Hispanic patients. If DM is diagnosed in the first trimester or early second trimester with an HbA1C of 6.5% or greater, a fasting glucose of 126 mg/dL or greater, or a 2-hour glucose level of 200 mg/dL or greater with a 75-g OGTT, it is considered pregestational DM (ACOG, 2018b). Preexisting DM becomes more difficult to control in the second and third trimesters due to placental hormones. It requires close monitoring and insulin adjustment. Complications of hyperglycemia include spontaneous abortion, fetal malformations, fetal macrosomia, fetal death, neonatal respiratory distress syndrome, polycythemia, organomegaly, electrolyte imbalances, and hyperbilirubinemia (ACOG, 2018b). The complications are mediated with glucose control. Diet, exercise, and medications are instrumental in glucose control. Optimal fasting and postprandial levels are the same for both GDM and preexisting DM. The goal is to achieve euglycemia without hypoglycemia. Diabetic ketoacidosis (DKA) is a concern with blood glucose levels over 200 mg/dL. DKA is a life-threatening emergency presenting clinically with abdominal pain, nausea, vomiting, and altered sensorium. Diagnosis is based on laboratory findings, including a low arterial pH, a low serum bicarbonate level (<15 mEq/L), an elevated anion gap, and positive serum ketones. FHR pattern changes include minimal variability and late decelerations that resolve, as with the improvement of maternal condition with IV insulin and IV fluids. Maternal risks with uncontrolled diabetes include worsening of retinopathy and nephropathy, risk for end-organ damage, hypertensive disorders, uteroplacental insufficiency, risk for acute myocardial infarction, medically indicated preterm delivery, polyhydramnios, shoulder dystocia, and increased risk of Cesarean delivery. Baseline evaluation of renal function testing and baseline EKG are recommended prior to pregnancy, especially with long-standing DM. Increased antepartum fetal surveillance and serial fetal growth monitoring are recommended to assess for complications related to uncontrolled DM such as macrosomia, polyhydramnios, and frequent fetal assessment due to the risk of stillbirth. Additionally, due to the risk of congenital anomalies with preexisting DM, a targeted ultrasound and fetal echocardiography may be indicated (ACOG, 2018b). Treatment of preexisting DM is the same as treatment for GDM, with insulin as the preferred treatment method. During the intrapartum period, IV insulin may be required to manage glucose levels.

MATERNAL SYSTEMIC LUPUS ERYTHEMATOSUS

SLE is one of the more common autoimmune diseases in young patients and can affect any organ in the body. SLE is a leading cause of death in young patients, with a higher rate of death in African American and Hispanic patients (Yen & Singh, 2018). Morbidity and mortality are related to the development of end-organ damage over time. SLE affects primarily women and presents in puberty or young adulthood. It is caused by genetic, environmental, and hormonal factors. Common alleles lead to an overactive immune system. Environmental UV light exposure, infections, smoking, pollutants, mercury, and insecticides may cause SLE and SLE flares (Petri, 2020). Estrogen is thought to play a role in the causation of SLE.

> ### Clinical Pearl
>
> SLE is an autoimmune disease leading to end-organ damage over time.

SLE is a diagnosis of exclusion based on clinical and laboratory findings. The diagnosis is difficult due to overlapping clinical presentations and laboratory findings with other autoimmune diseases. A rheumatologist, a dermatologist, and specialists depending on organ involvement are often needed for diagnosis. Laboratory tests include antinuclear antibody, antiphospholipid antibody, anti-dsDNA, and anti-Sm. Clinical presentations include cutaneous symptoms, joint involvement, nephritis, pleurisy, pericarditis, and various neurologic and hematologic manifestations (Petri, 2020). Pleurisy is sustained pain at the end of every breath. Pericarditis is characterized as pain when lying down or leaning forward. Neurologic involvement with SLE includes seizures or psychosis and, in serious manifestations, encephalopathy or coma. Hematologic manifestations of SLE include anemia, leukopenia, thrombocytopenia, increased erythrocyte sedimentation rate, and presence of autoantibodies. Anti-Ro/SS-A antibodies and anti-LA/SS-B antibodies are sometimes found with SLE. They cause additional concern in pregnancy because they can cross the placenta and bind to the fetal cardiac conduction system, leading to fetal congenital heart block (Petri, 2020).

Clinical Pearl

Anti-Ro/SS-A antibodies and anti-LA/SS-B antibodies are sometimes found with SLE and can cause fetal congenital heart block.

Treatment for SLE primarily includes prevention of SLE flares secondary to exposures. This includes avoidance of diseases by obtaining vaccinations and lifestyle modifications such as avoiding UV light exposure, avoiding stress, exercising, and maintaining a healthy diet. Pharmacologic treatments may be indicated; however, the risks of fetal exposure should be considered. Pharmacologic treatment is individualized based on the organ involvement and the patient's specific manifestations of SLE.

Pregnancy can cause or worsen lupus nephritis secondary to SLE. There is increased maternal mortality and morbidity with SLE. Those with antiphospholipid antibodies are at additional risk for thrombosis requiring anticoagulant therapy during pregnancy (ACOG, 2012). Adverse pregnancy outcomes include preterm birth, premature rupture of membranes, preeclampsia, and fetal growth restriction. Antiphospholipid antibodies common with SLE increase neonatal risk of stillbirth and miscarriage (Petri, 2020).

ACUTE FATTY LIVER OF PREGNANCY

Acute fatty liver of pregnancy (AFLP) is a rare but potentially fatal obstetric complication. AFLP is associated with severe maternal morbidities and a maternal mortality as high as 80% if supportive measures and delivery are not implemented (Nelson et al., 2021). AFLP typically presents in the third trimester and requires delivery and supportive care. It is characterized by a coagulation defect with hepatic and renal dysfunction. After delivery, the coagulation deficiency typically resolves in a few days, and renal and hepatic function returns to baseline.

Clinical Pearl

AFLP is characterized by a coagulation defect with hepatic and renal dysfunction associated with severe maternal morbidities and risk for maternal mortality.

Risk factors associated with AFLP include multifetal gestation, nulliparity, male fetus, fetal fatty acid oxidation disorders, obesity, DM, and hepatic disorders such as intrahepatic cholestasis. Preeclampsia may be associated with AFLP. Swansea criteria is used to diagnose AFLP but is not helpful for early diagnosis. The clinical presentation of AFLP is often nonspecific and can be confused with other obstetric complications. Common clinical findings with AFLP are hypertension, nausea, vomiting, abdominal pain, jaundice, gastrointestinal bleeding, and pruritus. Laboratory findings include elevated liver enzymes, hyperbilirubinemia, elevated white blood cell (WBC) count, serum creatinine consistent with acute kidney injury, low platelets, low glucose levels, and labs consistent with coagulopathy such as an elevated prothrombin time (PT) or low fibrinogen levels. DIC can also occur with AFLP. Some studies have reported that up to 80% of patients with AFLP meet diagnostic criteria for DIC. It can be difficult to differentiate AFLP from HELLP syndrome. Management of AFLP varies depending on the severity of the occurrence, ranging from mild metabolic and hematologic disturbances to hepatic encephalopathy, liver failure, and coagulopathy. Prompt recognition, supportive care, reversal of coagulopathy, expedited delivery, and a multidisciplinary care approach are key factors for management of AFLP and maternal survival (Nelson et al., 2021). Continuous fetal monitoring is important with the risk of maternal lactic acidosis and decreased uteroplacental blood flow that occurs with AFLP.

INTRAHEPATIC CHOLESTASIS OF PREGNANCY

Intrahepatic cholestasis of pregnancy (IHCP) presents with pruritus and is diagnosed by elevated total serum bile acid levels above 10 umol/L (Lee et al., 2021). Pruritus with IHCP is generalized with increased involvement of the palms of hands and soles of feet, which is worse at night. The pruritus is not associated with a rash other than possible excoriation from itching. IHCP typically presents later in the second and third trimesters of pregnancy. Increased levels of liver enzymes (transaminases) may also be seen but are not required for diagnosis. IHCP in pregnancy is a sign of underlying hepatic disease including a biliary tract disease or, less often, an autoimmune disease that is likely caused by environmental and hormonal factors with a genetic predisposition (Lee et al., 2021). In most cases, IHCP resolves after delivery.

> ### Clinical Pearl
>
> IHCP is diagnosed by elevated serum bile acids, presents as generalized pruritus with no accompanying rash, and increases the fetal risk of stillbirth.

Those with a history of liver, bile duct, and/or gallbladder disease are at higher risk for IHCP, and those with a history of IHCP are at increased risk for recurrence in a future pregnancy. Multiple gestations and advanced maternal age are also risk factors for IHCP (Lee et al., 2021).

Complications of IHCP in pregnancy include stillbirth, preeclampsia, fetal distress, meconium-stained amniotic fluid (MSAF), spontaneous or medically indicated preterm birth, and respiratory distress syndrome. The severity and presence of adverse outcomes correlate with the elevation of bile acids. Studies have shown that stillbirth rates are increased with total bile acids ≥40 umol/L; the highest risk is in those with total bile acids ≥100 umol/L. Bile acids activate myometrial oxytocin receptors, contributing to increased risk of spontaneous preterm birth (Lee et al., 2021).

Medications are used to decrease adverse outcomes by reducing the total bile acids and to reduce maternal symptoms. Ursodeoxycholic acid (UDCA) is recommended as first-line treatment for IHCP. Alternative drugs can be used when UDCA is contraindicated; these include S-adenosyl-methionine and cholestyramine. Oral antihistamines are often used for symptom treatment with pruritus. Topical antipruritic ointments are not usually beneficial because the itching is extensive.

The cause of stillbirth with IHCP is not clear; however, it is thought that the increased levels of bile acids cause fetal cardiac arrhythmias and placental vessel spasms leading to sudden fetal death (Ovadia et al., 2019). Antepartum fetal testing is recommended; however, due to the sudden nature of stillbirth with IHCP, the efficacy is not predictable. Timing of delivery is dependent on the risk of stillbirth with a higher total bile acid level and is individualized. Continuous EFM is recommended during labor due to the increased risk of stillbirth.

MATERNAL THYROID DISEASE

Pregnancy causes physiologic changes in maternal thyroid function. The thyroid volume increases later in pregnancy. Thyroid hormone levels fluctuate, and thyroid function adjusts throughout the pregnancy. Maternal thyroid hormones are important for fetal brain development and neonatal thyroid function.

Hyperthyroidism

Hyperthyroidism is characterized by low thyroid-stimulating hormone (TSH) levels and elevated free thyroxine (T_4) levels. Graves disease is the most common cause of overt hyperthyroidism. Clinical presentation includes nervousness, heart palpitations, tremors, insomnia, tachycardia, goiter, frequent stools, excessive sweating, heat intolerance, weight loss, and hypertension (ACOG, 2020b). Ophthalmopathy and dermopathy are seen with Graves disease.

Uncontrolled hyperthyroidism leads to increased risk for preeclampsia with severe features, maternal heart failure, and thyroid storm. Maternal thyroid storm is a rare, acute, and life-threatening condition with a high risk for maternal heart failure. It is caused by an excess of thyroid hormone and presents clinically with fever, tachycardia, cardiac dysrhythmia, and central nervous system dysfunction (ACOG, 2020b). The excessive thyroid hormones cause myocardial effects resulting in pulmonary hypertension from cardiomyopathy. Precipitating factors include preeclampsia, anemia, and sepsis. Urgent recognition, treatment of precipitating factors, and supportive care are needed for this critical but often reversible condition.

Clinical Pearl

Maternal thyroid storm is a rare, acute, and life-threatening condition with a high risk for maternal heart failure.

Fetal risk in uncontrolled hyperthyroidism includes low birth weight, miscarriage, stillbirth, and medically indicated preterm deliveries. Maternal antibodies common with hyperthyroidism cross the placenta and add a further risk of fetal thyrotoxicosis that manifests as fetal tachycardia and fetal growth restriction. A fetal goiter and fetal hydrops may be present with fetal thyrotoxicosis. Newborns should be followed by the pediatric provider due to risk of neonatal Graves disease or hyperthyroidism.

Hypothyroidism

Hypothyroidism is characterized by elevated TSH and low free T_4 levels. The glandular destruction by autoantibodies that is present with Hashimoto thyroiditis is the most common cause of hypothyroidism in pregnancy. Clinical presentation for hypothyroidism includes fatigue, edema, constipation, dry skin, hair loss, cold intolerance, muscle cramps, and weight gain (ACOG, 2020b). Goiter may be present more often in those with Hashimoto thyroiditis or in those with iodine deficiency (ACOG, 2020b). Maternal iodine intake is important for maternal and neonatal synthesis of T_4.

Untreated hypothyroidism can cause adverse pregnancy outcomes including miscarriage, preeclampsia, preterm birth, stillbirth, and placental abruption (ACOG, 2020b). Fetal adverse outcomes with untreated maternal hypothyroidism include low birth weight and impaired neuropsychological development of the newborn.

AMNIOTIC FLUID EMBOLISM

Amniotic fluid embolism is a rare but often fatal maternal condition in pregnancy. Timely recognition and appropriate supportive treatment are imperative in improving maternal and perinatal outcomes. The pathophysiology of an amniotic fluid embolism involves complex events causing a proinflammatory systemic response due to the introduction of fetal-material (amniotic) fluid into the maternal circulation. The maternal-fetal interface is disrupted, leading to increased levels of pulmonary vasoconstrictors and causing acute respiratory failure with severe hypoxemia and acute right ventricular failure. Right ventricular failure causes hemodynamic collapse and decreases the left-sided cardiac output, causing pulmonary edema and systemic hypotension. Amniotic fluid also activates factor VII in the clotting cascade and activates platelets, leading to DIC in over 80% of cases. The hemorrhages associated with DIC additionally contribute to hemodynamic instability (Pacheco et al., 2016). A severe cardiac event often ensues, with a poor prognosis.

The clinical presentation is often a triad of sudden maternal hypoxia, hypotension, and coagulopathy occurring during labor and delivery. The diagnosis is based on clinical presentation and exclusion of other causes. A patient may experience a period of anxiety, a change in mental status, and a sense of doom prior to cardiac arrest. If an event occurs while in labor, the EFM often shows FHR decelerations, loss of FHR variability, and terminal bradycardia (Pacheco et al., 2016).

Clinical Pearl

Amniotic fluid embolism presents as a triad of sudden maternal hypoxia, hypotension, and coagulopathy occurring during labor and delivery.

Risk factors for amniotic fluid embolism include any situation where the patient could be exposed to fetal material such as an operative delivery (vaginally or Cesarean), placenta previa, placental abruption, and placenta accrete spectrum disorders. Risk factors include cervical lacerations, uterine rupture, eclampsia, polyhydramnios, and multiple-gestation pregnancies (SMFM et al., 2018). Management includes supportive measures such as advanced cardiopulmonary resuscitation, reversing coagulopathy, expedited delivery, and a multidisciplinary team approach for care.

MATERNAL CARDIAC ARREST

Maternal cardiac arrest is infrequent, occurring in approximately 1 in 30,000 pregnancies, but often fatal (Campbell & Sanson, 2009). Causes for maternal cardiac arrest include hemorrhage, amniotic fluid embolism, acute coronary syndrome, and venous thromboembolism. Management components include oxygenation, high-quality chest compressions, and expedited delivery. The shortest time from cardiac arrest to delivery enhances outcomes for the patient and fetus (ACOG, 2019b). Knowledge of the anatomic and physiologic changes of pregnancy is imperative for successful resuscitation efforts. Standard resuscitation efforts should be initiated with minor modifications, including left uterine displacement to relieve pressure on the inferior vena cava to allow for optimal cardiac return. No modifications are required for defibrillation other than removal of fetal monitors. It does not increase fetal risk.

Once fetal viability is confirmed by fetal heart tones, emergent Cesarean delivery should be considered if the fundus is at least at the level of the umbilicus to improve maternal condition. If the patient is stable, continuous fetal monitoring may be considered. If attempts at maternal resuscitation fail, consider immediate delivery via perimortem Cesarean delivery in the patient's current location. Perimortem Cesarean delivery should be performed no later than 4 minutes after initial maternal arrest. Deliveries occurring more than 5 minutes from the initial cardiac arrest are unlikely to result in a normal neonate. Delivery sometimes results in maternal recovery due to the release of vena cava compression and improved cardiac return (Campbell & Sanson, 2009).

CHORIOAMNIONITIS

Chorioamnionitis is an infection with inflammation of the amniotic fluid, placenta, fetus, fetal membranes, or decidua (ACOG, 2017a). Poor maternal and fetal outcomes can result, including maternal uterine infection, septicemia, and fetal distress. The infection can lead to damage to the placental vasculature and fetal hypoxia followed by fetal distress and asphyxia, acidosis, and risk of hypoxic-ischemic encephalopathy.

Chorioamnionitis is diagnosed primarily with clinical criteria. Clinical presentations include maternal fever (≥38°C or ≥100.2°F), maternal tachycardia (≥100 bpm), uterine tenderness, foul-smelling amniotic fluid, fetal tachycardia, and laboratory results including an increased WBC (≥15 × 10⁹/L; ACOG, 2017a). Bacteria from group B streptococcus colonization and urinary tract infections are often the culprit. Bacteria invading the lower genital tract ascend and infect the sterile amniotic cavity. Chorioamnionitis less commonly occurs by invasive procedures such as amniocentesis. Risk factors include prolonged rupture of membranes and frequent vaginal exams.

> ### Clinical Pearl
>
> Chorioamnionitis is diagnosed primarily with clinical criteria reflective of an infection, including maternal fever, maternal tachycardia, uterine tenderness, odiferous amniotic fluid, and fetal tachycardia. Laboratory results show increased WBC count.

Treatment includes IV antibiotics, antipyretics, and delivery. Delivery is indicated to decrease the risk to the fetus regardless of the gestational age. Pyrexia (fever) during labor has been shown to increase the risk of neonatal encephalopathy regardless of the etiology (Greenwell et al., 2012). The increased temperature can result in greater consumption of fetal oxygen. EFM findings with maternal fever include fetal tachycardia (≥160 bpm).

UTERINE RUPTURE

Uterine rupture is most often associated with labor after Cesarean delivery and occurs rarely with an unscarred uterus. Uterine rupture can be life threatening with serious morbidity and mortality to the patient and fetus. The causes of uterine rupture include previous scar on uterus, trauma, uterine anomaly, and weakness of the myometrium due to congenital disease or prolonged stress from uterotonic drugs (Gibbins et al., 2015).

The clinical presentation includes abdominal pain, FHR changes such as bradycardia, late or variable decelerations, loss of station of the presenting fetal part, uterine tenderness, cessation of contractions, change in uterus shape, and/or vaginal bleeding (ACOG, 2019c). Management includes expedited delivery and maternal support for blood loss.

▶ PLACENTA COMPLICATIONS

PLACENTAL ABRUPTION

Placental abruption is when the placenta separates from the uterine wall and complicates approximately 1% of births (Oyelese & Ananth, 2006). It can vary from minor separation to complete separation, presenting with minor bleeding and little clinical significance, to severe bleeding with fetal death and maternal morbidity. Risk factors include prior abruption, preeclampsia, chronic hypertension, chorioamnionitis, premature rupture of membranes, low birth weight, polyhydramnios, oligohydramnios, nutritional deficiency, cigarette smoking, thrombophilia, cocaine use, uterine leiomyomas, and trauma (Oyelese & Ananth, 2006). Clinical findings include sudden onset of abdominal pain, vaginal bleeding, uterine tenderness, back pain, FHR characteristics of interrupted oxygenation, frequent uterine contractions, or persistent uterine hypertonus. It can also be asymptomatic (Oyelese & Ananth, 2006). Placental ultrasound is used for diagnosis; however, it fails to detect approximately half of cases (Oyelese & Ananth, 2006).

Management depends on the severity of the abruption, fetal status, and gestational age. Monitoring the patient and fetus is critical. Uterine hypertonus, characterized by high-frequency, low-amplitude contractions, may be found with external monitoring in the presence of a placental abruption. The uterus may feel hard on palpation. FHR patterns showing fetal bradycardia, loss of FHR variability, persistent late decelerations, or a sinusoidal FHR pattern indicate fetal compromise and should prompt expedited delivery (Oyelese & Ananth, 2006).

▶ FETAL COMPLICATIONS

AMNIOTIC FLUID DISORDERS

Amniotic fluid is critical for a healthy pregnancy, providing a cushion for the fetus and umbilical cord. It expands the uterus and allows fetal growth and movement necessary for fetal neuromusculoskeletal development. It is also important for fetal lung development. Amniotic fluid starts as a transudate plasma accumulating from the fetus through its skin, from the pregnant patient across the uterine decidua, and from the placental surface (Cunningham et al., 2022a). Later in pregnancy, fetal urine becomes a major component of the amniotic fluid (Cunningham et al., 2022a). Uteroplacental sufficiency, maternal hydration, and sufficient fetal organ function all play a role in the production and maintenance of the amniotic fluid.

Oligohydramnios

Oligohydramnios is amniotic fluid volume that is less than expected. Diagnosis is based on ultrasound findings of an amniotic fluid index less than 5 cm or a single deepest pocket of less than 2 cm (ACOG, 2016). The cause of oligohydramnios can be maternal, placental, or fetal. Oligohydramnios can be caused by maternal conditions leading to uteroplacental insufficiency, medications, and diabetes insipidus. Placental abruption, twin-to-twin transfusion, and placental thrombosis can cause oligohydramnios. Fetal causes include chromosomal abnormalities, congenital abnormalities, fetal growth restriction, post-term pregnancy, ruptured membranes, and infection (Cunningham et al., 2022a). Oligohydramnios can also be idiopathic. The prognosis and management for oligohydramnios depend on the severity of the condition, cause, and fetal status. Amniotic fluid is necessary for fetal lung maturity, fetal movement, and prevention of umbilical cord compression. Prolonged oligohydramnios can cause fetal deformities and is associated with increased risk of fetal or neonatal death. Early onset of oligohydramnios in preterm pregnancy is associated with a poor prognosis (Cunningham et al., 2022a). Pregnancies complicated by idiopathic oligohydramnios are at risk for meconium aspiration syndrome, Cesarean birth due to an abnormal FHR pattern, and NICU admission (Rabie et al., 2017).

> **Clinical Pearl**
>
> Oligohydramnios is amniotic fluid volume of less than 5 cm or a single deepest pocket of less than 2 cm. It is associated with an increased risk of stillbirth.

Antepartum fetal testing is recommended when oligohydramnios is detected due to the risk of stillbirth, while timing of delivery is individualized. Variable decelerations are noted with cord compression, which is thought to occur with oligohydramnios; however, studies have shown that term patients undergoing induction with and without oligohydramnios did not have a statistically significant difference in FHR patterns (Rhoades et al., 2019).

POLYHYDRAMNIOS

Polyhydramnios, or hydramnios, is an increase in the volume of amniotic fluid above the expected volume. Polyhydramnios is diagnosed by ultrasound measurement of an amniotic fluid index greater than or equal to 24 cm or a single deepest pocket that is greater than or equal to 8 cm (Dashe et al., 2018), most often found in the third trimester. Clinical presentation includes a fundal height that is greater than expected for the gestational age. Most cases of mild polyhydramnios are idiopathic. The most common causes are maternal DM and fetal anomalies (Dashe et al., 2018). Other causes of polyhydramnios include congenital infection and alloimmunization. Pregnancies complicated by polyhydramnios have increased risks of macrosomia, fetal malpresentation, and Cesarean delivery. Polyhydramnios is categorized as mild, moderate, or severe based on the amniotic fluid volume (Table 5.2). The likelihood of a fetal abnormality is associated with more severe polyhydramnios (SMFM, 2018).

Table 5.2 Polyhydramnios

Category	Amniotic Fluid Index	Single Deepest Pocket
Mild	24.0 to 29.9 cm	8 to 11 cm
Moderate	30.0 to 34.9 cm	12 to 15 cm
Severe	≥35 cm	≥16 cm

Source: Society for Maternal-Fetal Medicine, Dashe, J., Pressman, E., & Hibbard, J. (2018). *SMFM consult series #46: Evaluation and management of polyhydrmanios. B2-B8.* https://doi.org/10.1016/j.ajog.2018.07.016

Management of polyhydramnios is individualized depending on the etiology and severity of the fluid volume excess. An amnioreduction is considered only in severe cases. Antepartum fetal surveillance is performed when uteroplacental insufficiency is at risk. The risk of a dysfunctional labor pattern and postpartum hemorrhage is higher with polyhydramnios (Dashe et al., 2018). FHR patterns among those with and without polyhydramnios do not differ (Odibo et al., 2016).

MULTIFETAL GESTATION

Multifetal gestation is referred to as twin, triplet, or more gestations. Twin gestations are the most common occurrence and thus are the focus of this section. The incidence of multifetal gestations is higher with increased maternal age and assisted reproductive technology (ACOG, 2021b). Twin gestation has increased the risk of fetal, infant, and maternal morbidity and mortality. Maternal risks include hyperemesis, GDM, HDPs, anemia, Cesarean delivery, and hemorrhage (ACOG, 2021b).

Fetal risks are dependent on the zygosity, amnionicity, and chorionicity of the pregnancy. Dizygotic twins, or twins resulting from two separately fertilized ovum, are at least risk. Monozygotic twins arise from the division of a single fertilized ovum. The timing of the division is directly related to the outcome and the number of amnions and chorions. If the zygote (fertilized ovum) divides in the first 72 hours, the result will be two separate embryos, two amnions, and two chorions. This is referred to as a monozygotic, dichorionic/diamnionic (di/di) twin gestation. The two placentas may become fused, making chorionicity difficult to determine. An early assessment by ultrasound in the pregnancy can help to distinguish the chorionicity. Zygotic division on days 4 to 8 results in a monozygotic, monochorionic/diamnionic (mono/di) twin gestation. Division by day 8 results in a monozygotic, monochorionic/monoamnionic (mono/mono) twin gestation. Division later results in conjoined twins (Figure 5.1; Cunningham et al., 2022b).

Monochorionic twins have increased risk of morbidity and mortality compared with dichorionic twins. Fetal risks include discordant fetal growth, twin-to-twin transfusion with monochorionic twins, and stillbirth. Monoamniotic twin gestations have a perinatal mortality rate from 12% to 23% and are monitored closely and delivered between 32 and 34 weeks' gestation (ACOG, 2021b). Antepartum fetal surveillance is recommended due to the increased rate of stillbirth and morbidity in twin pregnancy. Delivery timing depends on the chorionicity and comorbidities of the twin gestation. Delivery is recommended earlier in even the lowest-risk twin pregnancies, dichorionic/diamniotic gestations, due to an increased stillbirth risk compared with singleton pregnancies. Continuous fetal monitoring is recommended in labor. The recommendation for Cesarean delivery is individualized and based on comorbidities, fetal presentations, and chorionicity.

MECONIUM-STAINED AMNIOTIC FLUID

MSAF is the presence of meconium in the amniotic fluid. Several risk factors have been identified for MSAF, including post-term pregnancy, placental insufficiency, and maternal complications such as IHCP (Rawat et al., 2018). MSAF is thought to be from either fetal maturity or fetal distress (Mitchell & Chandraharan, 2018). As the fetal gastrointestinal tract matures, meconium is produced and can pass prior to delivery. A fetal vagal response to cord compression is thought to cause passage of meconium and could indicate fetal distress (Mitchell & Chandraharan, 2018). The risk of MSAF is meconium aspiration syndrome. Delivery of infants, including resuscitation measures, should follow the same principles regardless of the presence of MSAF (ACOG, 2017b).

FETAL GROWTH RESTRICTION

Fetal growth restriction is described as a fetus with an estimated fetal weight or abdominal circumference that is less than the 10th percentile for gestational age, identified by ultrasonography (ACOG, 2019d). Fetal growth restriction can be caused by maternal, fetal, or placental factors. Maternal causes include any chronic disorder that is associated with vascular disease—for example, hypertensive diseases and thrombophilia. Substance use is associated with increased risk of a fetus that is small for gestational age at birth. Maternal malnutrition, multifetal gestations, teratogen exposure, and infectious disease are also associated with fetal growth restriction (ACOG, 2019d). Fetal growth restriction is associated with both genetic and structural disorders. Placental abruption, placental infarction, circumvallate placenta, hemangioma, and chorioangiomas are associated with fetal growth restriction due to poor placental perfusion (ACOG, 2019d).

Fetal risks include stillbirth, neonatal death, neonatal hypoglycemia, respiratory distress, hyperbilirubinemia, hypothermia, intraventricular hemorrhage, necrotizing enterocolitis, sepsis, and seizures in the neonate. Chromosomal abnormalities are more often a factor with the presence of fetal growth restriction with fetal structural abnormalities.

Due to the risk of stillbirth, antenatal surveillance is recommended. The timing of delivery depends on the severity of the fetal growth restriction and the fetal status. Fetal growth restriction is associated with fewer accelerations, a higher risk of decelerations, and an increased risk of late decelerations in the second stage of labor (Epplin et al., 2015). Continuous fetal monitoring is recommended during labor.

FETAL ANEMIA

Fetal anemia is a rare but possibly fatal risk to the fetus. Red blood cell alloimmunization is the most common cause of fetal anemia in the United States, and maternal infection from parvovirus is also a common cause. Other causes include inherited conditions, genetic metabolic disorders, fetal blood loss, and infection. Down syndrome is associated with fetal anemia. Diagnosis for fetal anemia is a hemoglobin that is more than two standard deviations below the mean according to gestational age (Mari et al., 2015). Severe anemia can lead to fetal hydrops and death. Fetal hydrops is accumulation of fluid in the fetal soft tissues and serous cavities. This is caused by an imbalance of regulation of the fluid moving from the vascular system to the interstitial spaces. It is caused by an underlying

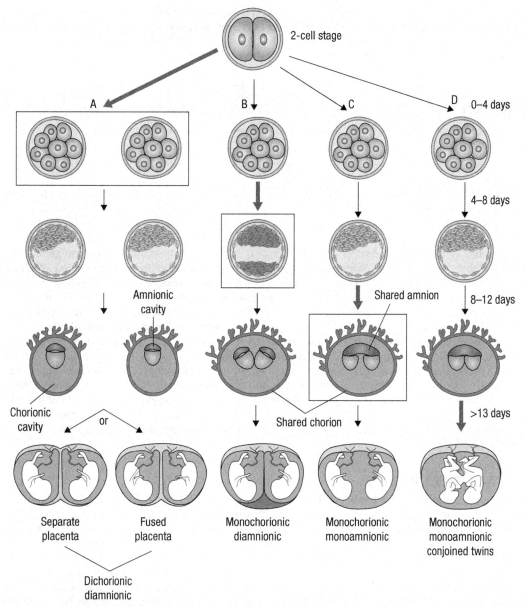

Figure 5.1 Mechanism of monozygotic twinning. Black boxing and thick arrows in columns A, B, and C indicate timing of division. **(A)** At 0 to 4 days postfertilization, an early conceptus may divide into two. Division at this early stage creates two chorions and two amnions (dichorionic, diamnionic). Placentas may be separate or fused. **(B)** Division between 4 and 8 days leads to formation of a blastocyst with two separate embryoblasts (inner cell masses). Each embryoblast will form its own amnion within a shared chorion (monochorionic, diamnionic). **(C)** Between 8 and 12 days, the amnion and amnionic cavity form above the germinal disc. Embryonic division leads to two embryos with a shared amnion and shared chorion (monochorionic, monoamnionic). **(D)** Differing theories explain conjoined twin development. One describes an incomplete splitting of one embryo into two. The other describes fusion of a portion of one embryo from a monozygotic pair onto the other.

Source: Adapted from Cunningham, F. G., Leveno, K. J., Bloom, S. L., Spong, C., & Dashe, J. (Eds.). (2014). *Williams Obstetrics*, (24th ed.). McGraw-Hill.

pathologic process, often severe fetal anemia leading to high-output cardiac failure and activation of red blood cells outside the bone marrow. This results in liver dysfunction, lymphatic dysfunction, and renal dysfunction, reducing osmotic pressure. Fetal hydrops is diagnosed with two or more abnormal fetal fluid collections identified on ultrasonography (Norton et al., 2015).

Clinical Pearl

Red blood cell alloimmunization and maternal infection from parvovirus are the most common causes of fetal anemia.

Red blood cell alloimmunization occurs when maternal antibodies cross the placenta and leads to hemolysis if the fetus is positive for the specific erythrocyte surface antigen. The antibody attacks the antigen, leading to hemolysis, called hemolytic disease of the newborn. Maternal alloimmunization occurs from sensitization to foreign erythrocyte surface antigens through blood transfusion or fetal-maternal hemorrhage during delivery, trauma, miscarriage, abortion, ectopic pregnancy, or invasive obstetric procedures (Norton et al., 2015). Rh(D) immune globulin decreases the risk of Rh(D) alloimmunization. However, Rh(D) immune globulin is not protective of other alloantibodies. Other Rh blood group antigens and atypical antigens can also cause a sensitization leading to maternal antibodies.

Parvovirus can cross the placenta and inhibits erythropoiesis in the fetus, resulting in anemia. The risk to the fetus is greatest prior to 20 weeks' gestation. Anemia in this case is transient but in some severe cases may require fetal intravascular transfusion (Norton et al., 2015). Twin-to-twin transfusion can also cause fetal anemia, leaving the donor twin deficient.

The management of fetal anemia is dependent on the cause and severity. Monitoring of maternal laboratory values, antepartum fetal surveillance, and ultrasound evaluation for the presence of fetal hydrops plays a role in the management decisions. If a fetus has significant risk of fetal anemia based on antepartum monitoring, a fetal blood sample and intrauterine fetal transfusion can be administered. Late decelerations and sinusoidal FHR patterns are increased with fetal anemia (Kariniemi, 1982).

FETAL HEART BLOCK

Congenital complete heart block (CCHB) is a third-degree fetal heart block, involves complete atrioventricular (AV) dissociation secondary to the disruption of the AV node, and results in significant fetal bradycardia with a heart rate of 40 to 90 beats per minutes (Pruetz et al., 2019). Maternal risk factors include metabolic disease, medication, viral infections, and autoantibodies. CCHB is associated with congenital heart anomalies such as complete AV canal defects. The current hypotheses for the cause of maternal antibodies specific for Ro-SSA and La-SSB leading to CCHB involves a pathway of inflammation leading to fibrosis and scarring of the fetal conduction system (Pruetz et al., 2019). Fetal echocardiography is the standard method for diagnosing fetal bradyarrhythmia. The goal of treatment is to identify early signs of fetal heart block and prevent progression to higher degrees of AV block and fetal hydrops while decreasing overall deterioration (Pruetz et al., 2019). Pharmacotherapy with corticosteroids is used to reduce the inflammatory response that causes damage in the early stages of fetal heart block. Third-degree fetal heart block is nonreversible. FHR patterns with CCHB reveal persistent bradycardia. Management by specialists is indicated.

▶ KEY POINTS

- ■ Diagnostic criteria for gestational hypertension include a systolic blood pressure ≥140 mmHg or a diastolic blood pressure ≥90 mmHg on two occasions 4 hours apart after 20 weeks' gestation with a previously normal blood pressure.
- ■ Preeclampsia diagnosis is made when a patient who meets criteria for gestational hypertension also has proteinuria (>300 mg per 24-hour urine collection, protein creatinine ratio of .3 or more, or a dipstick reading of 2+ if no other quantitative methods are available).
- ■ Severe-range blood pressures, or systolic blood pressure ≥160 mmHg, or diastolic blood pressure ≥110 mmHg should be diagnosed as preeclampsia with severe features.

- Severe features include blood pressures in the severe-range levels, thrombocytopenia less than 100×10^9/L, impaired liver function with liver enzymes more than twice the upper limit of normal or severe persistent right upper quadrant pain or epigastric pain, renal insufficiency with a serum creatinine >1.1 mg/dL or doubling, pulmonary edema, new-onset headache unresponsive to medications, or visual disturbances.
- Antihypertensive agents should be administered within 30 to 60 minutes with persistent (15 minutes or more) severe acute-onset hypertension.
- Eclampsia is a convulsive symptom of HDP. It is characteristic of severe disease. Convulsions are new-onset, tonic-clonic, focal or multifocal seizures in the absence of other causes such as epilepsy, cerebral arterial ischemia and infarction, drugs, or intracranial hemorrhages.
- Magnesium sulfate is considered first-line for prevention of eclampsia and is also used in the presence of eclampsia to prevent recurrent convulsions.
- Fetal risks include macrosomia, neonatal hypoglycemia, hyperbilirubinemia, polyhydramnios, shoulder dystocia, birth trauma, and stillbirth. Adequately controlling GDM in pregnancy reduces maternal and fetal risk factors.
- Type 1 pregestational DM is caused by an autoimmune process that destroys the pancreatic beta cells, requiring insulin therapy. Type 1 DM is frequently seen earlier in life and carries increased risk of development of vascular, renal, and neuropathic complications.
- Type 2 DM is due to peripheral insulin resistance, insulin deficiency, and obesity. It is more common later in life.
- SLE is an autoimmune disease leading to end-organ damage over time. Anti-Ro/SS-A antibodies and anti-LA/SS-B antibodies sometimes found with SLE can cause fetal congenital heart block.
- AFLP is characterized by a coagulation defect, with hepatic and renal dysfunction associated with severe maternal morbidities and risk for maternal mortality.
- IHCP is diagnosed by elevated serum bile acids, presents as generalized pruritus with no accompanying rash, and increases the fetal risk of stillbirth.
- Hyperthyroidism is characterized by low TSH levels and elevated free T_4 levels. It clinically presents with nervousness, heart palpitations, tremors, insomnia, tachycardia, goiter, frequent stools, excessive sweating, heat intolerance, weight loss, and hypertension.
- Hypothyroidism is characterized by elevated TSH and low free T_4 levels. Clinical presentations include fatigue, edema, constipation, dry skin, hair loss, cold intolerance, muscle cramps, weight gain, and goiter.
- Amniotic fluid embolism presents as a triad of sudden maternal hypoxia, hypotension, and coagulopathy occurring during labor and delivery from an inflammatory response to fetal material (amniotic fluid) in maternal circulation.
- The clinical presentation of uterine rupture includes abdominal pain, FHR changes such as bradycardia, late or variable decelerations, loss of station of the presenting fetal part, uterine tenderness, cessation of contractions, change in uterus shape, and vaginal bleeding.
- Polyhydramnios is diagnosed by ultrasound measurement of an amniotic fluid index greater than or equal to 24 cm or a single deepest pocket that is greater than or equal to 8 cm. Most mild cases are idiopathic, and severe polyhydramnios is associated with fetal abnormalities.
- Red blood cell alloimmunization and maternal infection from parvovirus are the most common causes of fetal anemia. Severe fetal anemia can lead to fetal hydrops and fetal death.
- The goal of treatment with fetal heart block is to identify early signs of fetal heart block and prevent progression to higher degrees of AV block and fetal hydrops, while decreasing deterioration.

CASE STUDY

Amy is 41-year-old G4P1213 patient presenting to the hospital at 36 weeks and 4 days' gestation with blood pressure of 146/92 mmHg. The pregnancy is complicated by chronic hypertension, GDM, and polyhydramnios. The patient reports regular contractions every 1 to 5 minutes, lasting 20 to 60 seconds for the last hour; states that her "water broke"; and reports a large amount of clear fluid leaking 15 minutes before arrival at the hospital. The patient reports uterine tenderness and vaginal bleeding. The EFM tracing is shown in the following.

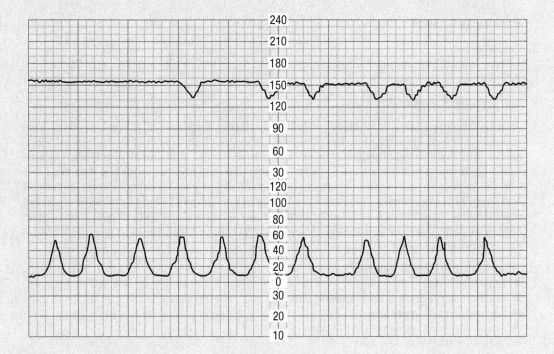

Answer the following, and then see the Case Study Answers for correct answers.

1. Baseline FHR: _____

2. Variability: _____

3. Accelerations: Present or absent?

4. Decelerations:
   a. Early: Present or absent?
   b. Variable: Present or absent?
   c. Late: Present or absent?
   d. Prolonged: Present or absent?

5. Contractions:
   a. Frequency: _____
   b. Duration: _____

6. Interpretation: Category: _____

7. Discuss the most likely physiologic rationale for the observed tracing given the clinical scenario.

8. List the priority physiologic goals for the observed tracing.

(See answers next page.)

CASE STUDY ANSWERS

1. Baseline FHR: 155 bpm

2. Variability: Minimal

3. Accelerations: Absent

4. Decelerations:
  a. Early: Absent
  b. Variable: Absent
  c. Late: Present
  d. Prolonged: Absent

5. Contractions:
  a. Frequency: q1 to 2 minutes
  b. Duration: 50 to 60 seconds

6. Interpretation: Category II

7. Placental abruption is the most likely rationale. Risk factors for placental abruption include prior abruption, preeclampsia, chronic hypertension, chorioamnionitis, premature rupture of membranes, low birth weight, polyhydramnios, oligohydramnios, nutritional deficiency, cigarette smoking, thrombophilia, cocaine use, uterine leiomyomas, and trauma (Oyelese & Ananth, 2006). Clinical findings include sudden onset of abdominal pain, vaginal bleeding, uterine tenderness, back pain, FHR characteristics of interrupted oxygenation, frequent uterine contractions, or persistent uterine hypertonus. It can also be asymptomatic (Oyelese & Ananth, 2006). Uterine hypertonus with high-frequency, low-amplitude contractions may be found with external monitoring in the presence of a placental abruption.

8. The priority goals are as follows:
- Expedite delivery
- Maintain appropriate level of uterine activity
- Maximize fetal oxygenation
- Maximize uteroplacental blood flow
- Maximize umbilical cord flow

FHR patterns showing fetal bradycardia, loss of FHR variability, persistent late decelerations, or a sinusoidal FHR pattern indicate fetal compromise and should prompt expedited delivery (Oyelese & Ananth, 2006). The fetal status suggests fetal hypoxia, and expectant management and labor augmentation are not recommended. The patient's presentation does not suggest normal labor or reassuring fetal status.

KNOWLEDGE CHECK: CHAPTER 5

1. A clinician is reviewing the chart of a patient who has been admitted for labor. They notice that the patient's initial blood pressure was 150/82 mmHg 6 hours ago. The patient's current blood pressure is 145/91. The patient denies vision disturbances, right upper quadrant pain, and headaches. The epidural was placed 2 hours ago, and the patient reports 0/10 pain. This patient meets criteria for:
   A) Gestational hypertension
   B) Preeclampsia with severe features
   C) Preeclampsia without severe features

2. A patient with preeclampsia with severe features on a titration of IV magnesium sulfate is in labor and desires an epidural. The anesthesia provider requests a 2-liter fluid bolus prior to the epidural placement. The clinician is concerned and wants to discuss the fluid bolus with the anesthesia provider. This extra caution is related to risk for:
   A) Pulmonary edema
   B) Seizures
   C) Thrombocytopenia

3. Symptoms of preeclampsia are related to the underlying pathology of the condition. Which is a cause for right upper quadrant pain that clinically presents with preeclampsia?
   A) Cerebral involvement
   B) Elevated perfusion pressure and hypertensive encephalopathy
   C) Hepatic cell edema

4. Antepartum testing with ultrasonography is used for fetal surveillance with preeclampsia to assess for:
   A) Fetal growth restriction
   B) Oligohydramnios
   C) Oligohydramnios and fetal growth restriction

5. During an eclamptic seizure, a fetal heart rate (FHR) tracing is likely to show:
   A) FHR baseline change
   B) Moderate variability with accelerations
   C) Prolonged late decelerations

6. A pregnant patient presents to the hospital with a sudden-onset severe headache, blood pressure of 162/90 mmHg, and 15 minutes later a blood pressure of 160/112 mmHg. This patient meets criteria for:
   A) Gestational hypertension
   B) Preeclampsia with severe features
   C) Preeclampsia without severe features

(See answers next page.)

1. A) Gestational hypertension

Diagnostic criteria for gestational hypertension include a systolic blood pressure ≥140 mmHg or a diastolic blood pressure ≥90 mmHg on two occasions 4 hours apart after 20 weeks' gestation with a previously normal blood pressure. The diagnosis of preeclampsia is made when a patient who meets criteria for gestational hypertension also has proteinuria (>300 mg per 24-hour urine collection, protein creatinine ratio of .3 or more, or a dipstick reading of 2+ if no other quantitative methods are available). A diagnosis of preeclampsia can be made without proteinuria with gestational hypertension and a new onset of one of the following: thrombocytopenia, renal insufficiency, impaired liver function, pulmonary edema, or new-onset headache unresponsive to medications and not accounted by an alternative diagnosis or visual disturbances. A patient with severe-range blood pressures, a systolic blood pressure ≥160 mmHg, or a diastolic blood pressure ≥110 mmHg should be diagnosed with preeclampsia with severe features.

2. A) Pulmonary edema

Patients with preeclampsia have hemoconcentration; they do not have the same increase in blood volume as in a normal pregnancy. Several vasodilators and vasoconstrictive agents interact, resulting in vasospasms. Patients with preeclampsia have hyperdynamic ventricular function and low pulmonary capillary wedge pressure. The pulmonary capillary wedge pressure increases significantly with excessive IV fluids and puts the patient at risk for pulmonary edema.

3. C) Hepatic cell edema

Liver dysfunction can occur due to periportal and focal parenchymal necrosis, hepatic cell edema, or Glisson capsule distension. Severe persistent right upper quadrant or epigastric pain unresolved with medications is due to liver involvement. New-onset headaches unresponsive to medications and visual disturbances are due to cerebral involvement. Headaches are thought to be caused by cerebral edema, elevated perfusion pressure, and hypertensive encephalopathy.

4. C) Oligohydramnios and fetal growth restriction

Preeclampsia fetal risks are associated with impaired uteroplacental blood flow resulting from placental dysfunction that limits the blood flow to the uteroplacental unit, causing ischemia. Clinical manifestations from uteroplacental ischemia include fetal growth restriction, stillbirth, oligohydramnios (low amniotic fluid), placental abruption, and findings on antepartum surveillance that are suggestive of fetal hypoxia.

5. C) Prolonged late decelerations

During an eclamptic seizure, the FHR pattern usually shows prolonged FHR decelerations and sometimes fetal bradycardia. Maternal hypoxia is the likely cause of the recurrent decelerations, tachycardia, and reduced variability often seen after a seizure. Maternal stabilization often normalizes the fetal tracing, and delivery is recommended only after the patient is hemodynamically stabilized. An FHR baseline change and moderate variability with accelerations are not suggestive of fetal hypoxia.

6. B) Preeclampsia with severe features

Severe features in preeclampsia include blood pressure in the severe-range levels, thrombocytopenia less than 100×10^9/L, impaired liver function with liver enzymes more than twice the upper limit of normal, severe persistent right upper quadrant pain or epigastric pain, renal insufficiency with a serum creatinine of more than 1.1 mg/dL, pulmonary edema, new-onset headache unresponsive to medications, and visual disturbances. A patient with severe-range blood pressures, or systolic blood pressure ≥160 mmHg, or diastolic blood pressure ≥110 mmHg should be diagnosed with preeclampsia with severe features.

7. Which statement is *true* regarding the pathophysiology of gestational diabetes mellitus (GDM)?
   A) GDM is caused by an autoimmune process that destroys the pancreatic beta cells, requiring insulin therapy
   B) GDM is caused by peripheral insulin resistance and insulin deficiency
   C) GDM is due to placental hormones causing mild postprandial elevated glucose levels, carbohydrate intolerance, and maternal inadequate insulin response

8. Fetal risks related to gestational diabetes include:
   A) Fetal macrosomia
   B) Precipitous labor
   C) Premature rupture of membranes

9. Which of the following interventions is recommended for patients with gestational diabetes?
   A) Delayed delivery
   B) Increased antepartum surveillance
   C) Routine antepartum surveillance

10. Which statement is *true* regarding type 2 diabetes mellitus (DM)?
    A) It is an autoimmune process that destroys pancreatic beta cells
    B) It is due to peripheral insulin resistance and insulin deficiency
    C) It usually presents early in life

11. A patient with systemic lupus erythematosus (SLE) is positive for anti-Ro/SS-A antibodies and anti-LA/SS-B antibodies. The fetal heart rate (FHR) tracing shows persistent fetal bradycardia in the 80s, indicating which pathologic condition that can result from the antibodies?
    A) Fetal growth restriction
    B) Fetal heart block
    C) Transposition of the great vessels

12. Antepartum fetal testing shows a fetal goiter, fetal growth restriction, and fetal tachycardia. Which fetal risk is associated with these findings with maternal hyperthyroidism with maternal thyroid antibodies?
    A) Fetal euthyroid
    B) Fetal hypothyroidism
    C) Fetal thyrotoxicosis

13. Which laboratory findings are most commonly associated with hypothyroidism?
    A) Elevated thyroid-stimulating hormone (TSH) levels and elevated free thyroxine (T_4) levels
    B) Elevated TSH levels and low free T_4 levels
    C) Low TSH levels and elevated T_4 levels

14. A patient with uncontrolled hyperthyroidism may have which clinical presentation?
    A) Fatigue, dry skin, cold intolerance, hair loss, and constipation
    B) Frequent stools, muscle cramps, goiter, weight loss, and edema
    C) Heart palpitations, nervousness, tachycardia, and heat intolerance

15. A patient presents to the obstetric ED at 38 weeks' gestation complaining of abdominal pain, nausea, vomiting, and itching. The blood pressure is 156/98 mmHg. The patient has jaundice and is not contracting, and laboratory values indicate coagulopathy. The provider alerts the healthcare team and prepares for an expedited delivery. The most likely diagnosis is:
    A) Acute fatty liver of pregnancy (AFLP)
    B) Hepatitis B
    C) Preeclampsia with severe features

(See answers next page.)

7. C) GDM is due to placental hormones causing mild postprandial elevated glucose levels, carbohydrate intolerance, and maternal inadequate insulin response

Glucose uptake by the fetus and placenta causes fasting glucose levels to be lower in a normal pregnancy than in the nonpregnant state. Placental hormones cause mild postprandial elevated glucose levels and carbohydrate intolerance. In normal pregnancies, the maternal pancreas can increase insulin production to compensate for the elevated glucose levels. In GDM, the insulin response is inadequate. Type 1 pregestational diabetes mellitus (DM) is caused by an autoimmune process that destroys the pancreatic beta cells, requiring insulin therapy. Type 1 DM is frequently seen earlier in life and has increased risk of development of vascular, renal, and neuropathic complications. Type 2 DM is due to peripheral insulin resistance and insulin deficiency. It is more common later in life.

8. A) Fetal macrosomia

Fetal risks with gestational diabetes include macrosomia, neonatal hypoglycemia, hyperbilirubinemia, polyhydramnios, shoulder dystocia, birth trauma, and stillbirth. Premature rupture of membranes and precipitous labor are not risks with gestational diabetes.

9. B) Increased antepartum surveillance

Increased antepartum fetal surveillance and serial fetal growth monitoring are recommended with gestational diabetes to assess for complications related to uncontrolled diabetes, such as macrosomia, polyhydramnios, and risk of stillbirth.

10. B) It is due to peripheral insulin resistance and insulin deficiency

Type 2 DM is due to peripheral insulin resistance and insulin deficiency and more commonly occurs later in life. Type 1 DM is caused by an autoimmune process that destroys the pancreatic beta cells, requiring insulin therapy. Type 1 DM is frequently seen earlier in life and has an increased risk of development of vascular, renal, and neuropathic complications.

11. B) Fetal heart block

Anti-Ro/SS-A antibodies and anti-LA/SS-B antibodies are sometimes found with SLE. They cause additional concern in pregnancy because they can cross the placenta and bind to the fetal cardiac conduction system, leading to fetal congenital heart block.

12. C) Fetal thyrotoxicosis

Maternal antibodies common with hyperthyroidism cross the placenta and add a further risk of fetal thyrotoxicosis that manifests as fetal tachycardia and fetal growth restriction. A fetal goiter and fetal hydrops may be present with fetal thyrotoxicosis.

13. B) Elevated TSH levels and low free T_4 levels

Hypothyroidism is characterized by elevated TSH levels and low free T_4 levels. Hyperthyroidism is characterized by low TSH levels and elevated free T_4 levels.

14. C) Heart palpitations, nervousness, tachycardia, and heat intolerance

The clinical presentation of hyperthyroidism includes nervousness, heart palpitations, tremors, insomnia, tachycardia, goiter, frequent stools, excessive sweating, heat intolerance, weight loss, and hypertension. The clinical presentation of hypothyroidism includes fatigue, edema, constipation, dry skin, hair loss, cold intolerance, muscle cramps, and weight gain. Goiter may be present more often in those with Hashimoto thyroiditis or in those with iodine deficiency.

15. A) AFLP

AFLP typically presents in the third trimester. It is characterized by a coagulation defect with hepatic and renal dysfunction. Common clinical findings with AFLP are hypertension, nausea, vomiting, abdominal pain, jaundice, gastrointestinal bleeding, and pruritus. DIC can occur with AFLP. Management of AFLP varies depending on the severity of the occurrence, ranging from mild metabolic and hematologic disturbances to hepatic encephalopathy, liver failure, and coagulopathy. Prompt recognition, supportive care, reversal of coagulopathy, expedited delivery, and a multidisciplinary care approach are key factors for management of AFLP and maternal survival. Hepatitis B does not have a risk of coagulopathy, and the clinical criteria for preeclampsia with severe features has not been met by this patient.

16. A patient presents with generalized itching, worse at night, that is located on the palms of the hands and the soles of the feet. There is no associated rash. Which of the following laboratory values is consistent with intrahepatic cholestasis of pregnancy (IHCP)?
    A) Aspartate aminotransferase (AST) and alanine aminotransferase (ALT) elevated to more than twice the upper limit of normal
    B) Platelet count of less than 100×10^9/L
    C) Total serum bile acid levels above 10 umol/L

17. A patient with a first pregnancy at 39 weeks' gestation presents to the obstetric ED reporting a large gush of fluid 3 days ago. The patient reports continuing leakage of foul-smelling fluid. Temperature is 101.1°F (38.39°C), and maternal pulse is 118. The laboratory results reveal a white blood cell count (WBC) of 20×10^9/L. The fetal heart rate (FHR) baseline is 165 beats per minute (bpm) with moderate variability. The most likely diagnosis for this patient is:
    A) Chorioamnionitis
    B) Intrahepatic cholestasis of pregnancy (IHCP)
    C) Oligohydramnios

18. Which triad is most commonly seen with an amniotic fluid embolism?
    A) Maternal fever, maternal tachycardia, and elevated white blood cell count (WBC)
    B) Maternal hypoxia, hypotension, and coagulopathy
    C) Severe hypertension, pulmonary edema, and coagulopathy

19. A laboring patient desires a vaginal birth after having had a previous Cesarean delivery. Which findings lead the nurse to suspect uterine rupture?
    A) Frequent uterine contractions, vaginal bleeding, and abdominal pain
    B) Late decelerations, loss of station of the presenting part, and abdominal pain
    C) Variable decelerations, thick green-colored amniotic fluid, and maternal fever

20. A patient presents with sudden-onset abdominal pain, vaginal bleeding, back pain, and frequent uterine contractions. The fetal heart rate (FHR) is a category I tracing. The provider orders an ultrasound to assess the placenta. What diagnosis is the provider considering?
    A) Placenta previa
    B) Placental abruption
    C) Uterine rupture

21. Diagnosis of oligohydramnios is an ultrasound finding of:
    A) Amniotic fluid index less than 5 cm
    B) Single deepest pocket less than 3 cm
    C) Single deepest pocket less than 5 cm

22. Which of the following is *true* regarding polyhydramnios?
    A) Almost always caused by fetal anomalies
    B) Diagnosed by amniotic fluid index ≥24 cm
    C) Most often found in the second trimester

(*See answers next page.*)

16. C) Total serum bile acid levels above 10 umol/L

IHCP presents with pruritus and is diagnosed by elevated total serum bile acid levels above 10 umol/L. Pruritus with IHCP is generalized, with increased involvement of the palms of the hands and soles of the feet, and is worse at night. The pruritus is not associated with a rash other than possible excoriation from itching. Complications of IHCP in pregnancy include stillbirth, preeclampsia, fetal distress, MSAF, spontaneous or medically indicated preterm birth, and respiratory distress syndrome. The severity and presence of adverse outcomes correlate with the elevation of bile acids. Studies have shown that stillbirth rates are increased with total bile acids ≥40 umol/L, and the highest risk is in patients with total bile acids ≥100 umol/L. Bile acids activate myometrial oxytocin receptors, contributing to the increased risk of spontaneous preterm birth. Low platelets are not diagnostic for IHCP.

17. A) Chorioamnionitis

Chorioamnionitis is diagnosed primarily with clinical criteria. The increased temperature can result in greater consumption of fetal oxygen. EFM findings with maternal fever include fetal tachycardia (>160 bpm). Clinical presentations for chorioamnionitis include maternal fever (≥100.1°F or ≥38°C), maternal tachycardia (>100 bpm), uterine tenderness, odiferous amniotic fluid, and fetal tachycardia. Laboratory results will show an increased WBC ($>15 \times 10^9$/L). Oligohydramnios, low amniotic fluid, and IHCP are not clinically represented in this scenario.

18. B) Maternal hypoxia, hypotension, and coagulopathy

Amniotic fluid embolism is a rare but often fatal maternal condition in pregnancy. The pathophysiology of an amniotic fluid embolism involves complex events causing a proinflammatory systemic response due to the introduction of fetal material (amniotic fluid) into the maternal circulation. The clinical presentation is often a triad of sudden maternal hypoxia, hypotension, and coagulopathy occurring during labor and delivery. The patient may experience a period of anxiety, a change in mental status, and a sense of doom prior to the cardiac arrest.

19. B) Late decelerations, loss of station of the presenting part, and abdominal pain

The clinical presentation of uterine rupture includes abdominal pain, fetal heart rate (FHR) changes such as bradycardia, late or variable decelerations, loss of station of the presenting fetal part, uterine tenderness, cessation of contractions, change in uterus shape, and vaginal bleeding. Variable decelerations, thick green-colored amniotic fluid, and maternal fever could indicate chorioamnionitis. Frequent uterine contractions, vaginal bleeding, and abdominal pain are consistent with placental abruption.

20. B) Placental abruption

Clinical findings of placental abruption include sudden onset of abdominal pain, vaginal bleeding, uterine tenderness, back pain, FHR characteristics of interrupted oxygenation, frequent uterine contractions, and persistent uterine hypertonus, but it can also be asymptomatic. Ultrasonography examination of the placenta is used for diagnosis; however, it fails to detect approximately half of cases. The patient is not exhibiting signs of placenta previa or uterine rupture.

21. A) Amniotic fluid index less than 5 cm

Oligohydramnios is defined as amniotic fluid volume that is less than the expected volume. Diagnosis is based on ultrasound findings of an amniotic fluid index less than 5 cm or a single deepest pocket of less than 2 cm.

22. B) Diagnosed by amniotic fluid index ≥24 cm

Polyhydramnios, or hydramnios, is an increase in the volume of amniotic fluid above the expected volume. Polyhydramnios is diagnosed by ultrasound measurement of an amniotic fluid index ≥24 cm or a single deepest pocket that is ≥8 cm. It is most often found in the third trimester. Most cases of mild polyhydramnios are idiopathic. The most common causes are maternal diabetes mellitus (DM) and fetal anomalies. Pregnancies complicated by polyhydramnios have increased risks of macrosomia, fetal malpresentation, and Cesarean delivery. The risk of a dysfunctional labor pattern is higher with polyhydramnios. There is also an increased risk for postpartum hemorrhage.

23. In a multifetal gestation pregnancy, zygotic division in the first 72 hours is associated with which type of twin pregnancy?
    A) Monoamniotic/dichorionic
    B) Monoamniotic/monochorionic
    C) Diamniotic/dichorionic

24. Fetal growth restriction is associated with an increased risk of:
    A) Chorioamnionitis
    B) Prolonged accelerations
    C) Stillbirth

25. Which fetal heart rate (FHR) pattern is increased with fetal anemia?
    A) Late decelerations and sinusoidal FHR patterns
    B) Minimal variability and no increased risk found with decelerations
    C) Persistent fetal tachycardia and moderate variability

(See answers next page.)

23. C) Diamniotic/dichorionic

If the zygote divides in the first 72 hours, the result will be two separate embryos, two amnions, and two chorions. This is referred to as a monozygotic, dichorionic/diamnionic twin gestation.

24. C) Stillbirth

Fetal growth restriction is described as a fetus with an estimated fetal weight or abdominal circumference that is less than the 10th percentile for gestational age identified by ultrasonography. Fetal risks include stillbirth, neonatal death, neonatal hypoglycemia, respiratory distress, hyperbilirubinemia, hypothermia, intraventricular hemorrhage, necrotizing enterocolitis, sepsis, and seizures in the neonate. Fetal growth restriction is associated with fewer accelerations, a higher risk of decelerations, and an increased risk of late decelerations in the second stage of labor.

25. A) Late decelerations and sinusoidal FHR patterns

Late decelerations and sinusoidal FHR patterns are increased with fetal anemia.

▶ REFERENCES

Alanne, L., Bhide, A., Lantto, J., Huhta, H., Kokki, M., Haapsamo, M., Acharya, G., & Räsänen, J. (2021). Nifedipine disturbs fetal cardiac function during hypoxemia in a chronic sheep model at near term gestation. *American Journal of Obstetrics and Gynecology*, 225(5), 544.e1–544.e9. https://doi.org/10.1016/j.ajog.2021.04.228

Ambia, A. M., Wells, C. E., Yule, C. S., McIntire, D. D., & Cunningham, F. G. (2022). Fetal heart rate tracings associated with eclamptic seizures. *American Journal of Obstetrics and Gynecology*, 227(4), P622.e1–P622.e6. https://doi.org/10.1016/j.ajog.2022.05.058

American College of Obstetrics and Gynecology. (2012). ACOG practice bulletin no. 132: Antiphospholipid syndrome. *Obstetrics and Gynecology*, 120(6), 1514–1521. https://doi.org/10.1097/01.AOG.0000423816.39542.0f

American College of Obstetrics and Gynecology. (2016). Practice bulletin no. 175: Ultrasound in pregnancy. *Obstetrics and Gynecology*, 128(6), e241–e256. https://doi.org/10.1097/AOG.0000000000001815

American College of Obstetrics and Gynecology. (2017a). Committee opinion no. 712: Intrapartum management of intraamniotic infection. *Obstetrics & Gynecology*, 130(2), 490–492. https://doi.org/10.1097/AOG.0000000000002230

American College of Obstetrics and Gynecology. (2017b). Committee opinion no 689: Delivery of a newborn with meconium-stained amniotic fluid. *Obstetrics and Gynecology*, 129(3), e33–e34. https://doi.org/10.1097/AOG.0000000000001950

American College of Obstetrics and Gynecology. (2018a). ACOG practice bulletin no. 201: Pregestational diabetes mellitus. *Obstetrics and Gynecology*, 132(6), e228–e248. https://doi.org/10.1097/AOG.0000000000002960

American College of Obstetrics and Gynecology. (2018b). Practice bulletin no. 190: Gestational diabetes mellitus. *Obstetrics and Gynecology*, 131(2), e49–e64. https://doi.org/10.1097/AOG.0000000000002501

American College of Obstetrics and Gynecology. (2019a). ACOG practice bulletin no. 203: Chronic hypertension in pregnancy. *Obstetrics and Gynecology*, 133(1), e26–e50. https://doi.org/10.1097/AOG.0000000000003020

American College of Obstetrics and Gynecology. (2019b). ACOG practice bulletin no. 205: Vaginal birth after cesarean delivery. *Obstetrics and Gynecology*, 133(2), e110–e127. https://doi.org/10.1097/AOG.0000000000003078

American College of Obstetrics and Gynecology. (2019c). ACOG practice bulletin no. 212: Pregnancy and heart disease. *Obstetrics and Gynecology*, 133(5), e320–e356. https://doi.org/10.1097/AOG.0000000000003243

American College of Obstetrics and Gynecology. (2019d). ACOG practice bulletin no. 204: Fetal growth restriction. *Obstetrics and Gynecology*, 133(2), e97–e109. https://doi.org/10.1097/AOG.0000000000003070

American College of Obstetrics and Gynecology. (2020a). ACOG practice bulletin no. 222: Gestational hypertension and preeclampsia. *Obstetrics and Gynecology*, 135(6), e237–e260. https://doi.org/10.1097/AOG.0000000000003891

American College of Obstetrics and Gynecology. (2020b). ACOG practice bulletin no. 223: Thyroid disease in pregnancy. *Obstetrics and Gynecology*, 135(6), e261–e274. https://doi.org/10.1097/AOG.0000000000003893

American College of Obstetrics and Gynecology. (2021a). ACOG practice bulletin no. 229: Antepartum fetal surveillance. *Obstetrics and Gynecology*, 137(6), e116–e127. https://doi.org/10.1097/AOG.0000000000004410

American College of Obstetrics and Gynecology. (2021b). ACOG practice bulletin no. 231: Multifetal gestations: Twin, triplet, and higher-order multifetal pregnancies. *Obstetrics and Gynecology*, 137(6), e145–e162. https://doi.org/10.1097/AOG.0000000000004397

American Diabetes Association. (2021). Classification and diagnosis of diabetes: Standards of medical care in diabetes-2021. *Diabetes Care*, 44(Suppl 1), S15–S33. https://doi.org/10.2337/dc21-S002

American Diabetes Association Professional Practice Committee. (2022). Management of diabetes in pregnancy: Standards of medical care in diabetes—2022. *Diabetes Care*, 45(Suppl 1), S232–S243. https://doi.org/10.2337/dc22-S015

Cahill, A., Obido, A., Roehl, K., & Macones, G. (2013). Effect of growth restriction on intrapartum electronic fetal heart rate monitoring (EFM) patterns? *American Journal of Obstetrics and Gynecology, 208*(1), S314–S315. https://doi.org/10.1016/j.ajog.2012.10.086

Campbell, T. A., & Sanson, T. G. (2009). Cardiac arrest and pregnancy. *Journal of Emergencies, Trauma, and Shock, 2*(1), 34–42. https://doi.org/10.4103/0974-2700.43586

Cunningham, F., Leveno, K. J., Dashe, J. S., Hoffman, B. L., Spong, C. Y., & Casey, B. M. (Eds.). (2022a). Obstetrical imaging. In *Williams obstetrics* (26th ed.). McGraw Hill. https://access medicine.mhmedical.com/content.aspx?bookid=2977&sectionid=253983118

Cunningham, F., Leveno, K. J., Dashe, J. S., Hoffman, B. L., Spong, C. Y., & Casey, B. M. (Eds.). (2022b). Multifetal pregnancy. In *Williams obstetrics* (26th ed.). McGraw Hill. https://access medicine.mhmedical.com/content.aspx?bookid=2977&sectionid=263825445

Dashe, J. S., Pressman, E. K., & Hibbard, J. U. (2018). SMFM consult series 46: Evaluation and management of polyhydramnios. *American Journal of Obstetrics and Gynecology, 219*(4), B2–B8. https://doi.org/10.1016/j.ajog.2018.07.016

Egan, A. M., Dow, M. L., & Vella, A. (2020). A review of the pathophysiology and management of diabetes in pregnancy. *Mayo Clinic Proceedings, 95*(12), 2734–2746. https://doi.org/10.1016/j.mayocp.2020.02.019

Epplin, K. A., Tuuli, M. G., Odibo, A. O., Roehl, K. A., Macones, G. A., & Cahill, A. G. (2015). Effect of growth restriction on fetal heart rate patterns in the second stage of labor. *American Journal of Perinatology, 32*(9), 873–878. https://doi.org/10.1055/s-0034-1543954

Ford, N., Cox, S., Ko, J.,Ouyang, L., Romero, L., Colarusso, T., Ferre, C. D., Kroelinger, C. D., Hayes, D. K., & Barfield, W. D. (2022). Hypertensive disorders in pregnancy and mortality at delivery hospitalization—United States, 2017–2019. Centers for disease control. *MMWR Morbidity Mortality Weekly Report, 71*(17), 585–591. https://doi.org/10.15585/mmwr.mm7117a1

Gibbins, K. J., Weber, T., Holmgren, C. M., Porter, T. F., Varner, M. W., & Manuck, T. A. (2015). Maternal and fetal morbidity associated with uterine rupture of the unscarred uterus. *American Journal of Obstetrics and Gynecology, 213*(3), 382.e1–382.e6. https://doi.org/10.1016/j.ajog.2015.05.048

Graham, E. M., Petersen, S. M., Christo, D. K., & Fox, H. E. (2006). Intrapartum electronic fetal heart rate monitoring and the prevention of perinatal brain injury. *Obstetrics and Gynecology, 108*(3), 656–666. https://doi.org/10.1097/01.AOG.0000230533.62760.ef

Greenwell, E. A., Wyshak, G., Ringer, S. A., Johnson, L. C., Rivkin, M. J., & Lieberman, E. (2012). Intrapartum temperature elevation, epidural use, and adverse outcome in term infants. *Pediatrics, 129*(2), e447–e454. https://doi.org/10.1542/peds.2010-2301

Kariniemi, V. (1982). Fetal anemia and heart rate patterns. *Journal of Perinatal Medicine, 10*(3), 167–173. https://doi.org/10.1515/jpme.1982.10.3.167

Lee, R. H., Greenberg, M., Metz, T. D., & Pettker, C. M. (2021). Society for maternal-fetal medicine consult series #53: Intrahepatic cholestasis of pregnancy: Replaces consult #13, April 2011. *American Journal of Obstetrics and Gynecology, 224*(2), B2–B9. https://doi.org/10.1016/j.ajog.2020.11.002

Lisonkova, S., Razaz, N., Sabr, Y., Muraca, G. M., Boutin, A., Mayer, C., Joseph, K. S., & Kramer, M. S. (2020). Maternal risk factors and adverse birth outcomes associated with HELLP syndrome: A population-based study. *British Journal of Obstetrics and Gynaecology, 127*, 1189–1198.

Louis, J., Parchem, J., Vaught, A., Tesfalul, M., Kendle, A., & Tsigas, E. (2022). Society of maternal fetal medicine (SMFM) special report. Preeclampsia: A report and recommendations of the workshop of the society for maternal-fetal medicine and the preeclampsia foundation. *American Journal of Obstetrics and Gynecology, 227*(5), B2–B24. https://doi.org/10.1016/j.ajog.2022.06.038

Mari, G., Norton, M. E., Stone, J., Berghella, V., Sciscione, A. C., Tate, D., & Schenone, M. H. (2015). Society for maternal-fetal medicine (SMFM) clinical guideline 8: The fetus at risk for anemia—Diagnosis and management. *American Journal of Obstetrics and Gynecology, 212*(6), 697–710. https://doi.org/10.1016/j.ajog.2015.01.059

Mitchell, S. & Chandraharan, E. (2018). Meconium-stained amniotic fluid. *Obstetrics, Gynaecology & Reproductive Medicine, 28*(4), 120–124. https://doi.org/10.1016/j.ogrm.2018.02.004

Nelson, D. B., Byrne, J. J., & Cunningham, F. G. (2021). Acute fatty liver of pregnancy. *Obstetrics and Gynecology, 137*(3), 535–546. https://doi.org/10.1097/AOG.0000000000004289

Norton, M. E., Chauhan, S. P., & Dashe, J. S. (2015). Society for maternal-fetal medicine (SMFM) clinical guideline #7: Nonimmune hydrops fetalis. *American Journal of Obstetrics and Gynecology*, *212*(2), 127–139. https://doi.org/10.1016/j.ajog.2014.12.018

Odibo, I. N., Newville, T. M., Ounpraseuth, S. T., Dixon, M., Lutgendorf, M. A., Foglia, L. M., & Magann, E. F. (2016). Idiopathic polyhydramnios: Persistence across gestation and impact on pregnancy outcomes. *European Journal of Obstetrics, Gynecology, and Reproductive Biology*, *199*, 175–178. https://doi.org/10.1016/j.ejogrb.2016.02.018

Ovadia, C., Seed, P. T., Sklavounos, A., Geenes, V., Di Ilio, C., Chambers, J., Kohari, K., Bacq, Y., Bozkurt, N., Brun-Furrer, R., Bull, L., Estiú, M. C., Grymowicz, M., Gunaydin, B., Hague, W. M., Haslinger, C., Hu, Y., Kawakita, T., Kebapcilar, A. G., … Williamson, C. (2019). Association of adverse perinatal outcomes of intrahepatic cholestasis of pregnancy with biochemical markers: Results of aggregate and individual patient data meta-analyses. *Lancet*, *393*(10174), 899–909. https://doi.org/10.1016/S0140-6736(18)31877-4

Oyelese, Y., & Ananth, C. V. (2006). Placental abruption. *Obstetrics and Gynecology*, *108*(4), 1005–1016. https://doi.org/10.1097/01.AOG.0000239439.04364.9a

Pacheco, L. D., Saade, G., Hankins, G. D., & Clark, S. L. (2016). Amniotic fluid embolism: Diagnosis and management. *American Journal of Obstetrics and Gynecology*, *215*(2), B16–B24. https://doi.org/10.1016/j.ajog.2016.03.012

Petri, M. (2020). Systemic lupus erythematosus: Clinical updates in women's health care primary and preventive care review. *Obstetrics and Gynecology*, *136*(1), 226. https://doi.org/10.1097/AOG.0000000000003942

Pruetz, J. D., Miller, J. C., Loeb, G. E., Silka, M. J., Bar-Cohen, Y., & Chmait, R. H. (2019). Prenatal diagnosis and management of congenital complete heart block. *Birth Defects Research*, *111*(8), 380–388. https://doi.org/10.1002/bdr2.1459

Rabie, N., Magann, E., Steelman, S., & Ounpraseuth, S. (2017). Oligohydramnios in complicated and uncomplicated pregnancy: A systematic review and meta-analysis. *Ultrasound in Obstetrics & Gynecology: The Official Journal of the International Society of Ultrasound in Obstetrics and Gynecology*, *49*(4), 442–449. https://doi.org/10.1002/uog.15929

Rana, S., Lemoine, E., Granger, J. P., & Karumanchi, S. A. (2019). Preeclampsia: Pathophysiology, challenges, and perspectives. *Circulation Research*, *124*(7), 1094–1112. https://doi.org/10.1161/CIRCRESAHA.118.313276

Rawat, M., Nangia, S., Chandrasekharan, P., & Lakshminrusimha, S. (2018). Approach to infants born through meconium stained amniotic fluid: Evolution based on evidence? *American Journal of Perinatology*, *35*(9), 815–822. https://doi.org/10.1055/s-0037-1620269

Rhoades, J. S., Stout, M. J., Macones, G. A., & Cahill, A. G. (2019). Effect of oligohydramnios on fetal heart rate patterns during term labor induction. *American Journal of Perinatology*, *36*(7), 715–722. https://doi.org/10.1055/s-0038-1675152

Say, L., Chou, D., Gemmill, A., Tunçalp, Ö., Moller, A. B., Daniels, J., Gülmezoglu, A. M., Temmerman, M., & Alkema, L. (2014). Global causes of maternal death: A who systematic analysis. *The Lancet: Global Health*, *2*(6), e323–e333. https://doi.org/10.1016/S2214-109X(14)70227-X

Society for Maternal-Fetal Medicine, Dashe, J., Pressman, E., & Hibbard, J. (2018). *SMFM consult series #46: Evaluation and management of polyhydrmanios. B2-B8*. https://doi.org/10.1016/j.ajog.2018.07.016

Society for Maternal-Fetal Medicine Statement. (2022). Antihypertensive therapy for mild chronic hypertension in pregnancy—The chronic hypertension and pregnancy trial. *American Journal of Obstetrics and Gynecology*, *227*(2), 24–27. https://doi.org/10.1016/j.ajog.2022.04.011

U.S. Preventive Services Task Force, Davidson, K. W., Barry, M. J., Mangione, C. M., Cabana, M., Caughey, A. B., Davis, E. M., Donahue, K. E., Doubeni, C. A., Kubik, M., Li, L., Ogedegbe, G., Pbert, L., Silverstein, M., Stevermer, J., Tseng, C. W., & Wong, J. B. (2021). Screening for gestational diabetes: US preventive services task force recommendation statement. *Journal of the American Medical Association*, *326*(6), 531–538. https://doi.org/10.1001/jama.2021.11922

Usui, R., Matsubara, S., Ohkuchi, A., Kuwata, T., Watanabe, T., Izumi, A., & Suzuki, M. (2008). Fetal heart rate pattern reflecting the severity of placental abruption. *Archives of Gynecology and Obstetrics*, *277*(3), 249–253. https://doi.org/10.1007/s00404-007-0471-9

Waterman, E. J., Magee, L. A., Lim, K. I., Skoll, A., Rurak, D., & von Dadelszen, P. (2004). Do commonly used oral antihypertensives alter fetal or neonatal heart rate characteristics? A systematic review. *Hypertension in Pregnancy*, *23*(2), 155–169. https://doi.org/10.1081/PRG-120028291

Whelton, P., Carey, R., Aronow, W., Casey, D., Collins, K., Dennison Himmelfarb, C., DePalma, S., Gidding, S., Jamerson, K., Jones, D., MacLaughlin, E., Muntner, P., Ovbiagele, B., Smith, S., Spencer, C., Stafford, R., Taler, S., Thomas, R., Williams, K., Williamson, J., & Wright, J. (2018). 2017 ACC/AHA/AAPA/ABC/ACPM/AGS/APhA/ASH/ASPC/NMA/PCNA guidelines for the prevention, detection, evaluation, and management of high blood pressure in adults. *Hypertension*, *71*(19), e13–e115.

Xiao, M. Z. X., Whitney, D., Guo, N., Bentley, J., Shaw, G. M., Druzin, M. L., & Butwick, A. J. (2022). Trends in eclampsia in the United States, 2009–2017: A population-based study. *Journal of Hypertension*, *40*(3), 490–497. https://doi.org/10.1097/HJH.0000000000003037

Yen, E. Y., & Singh, R. R. (2018). Brief report: Lupus—An unrecognized leading cause of death in young females: A population-based study using nationwide death certificates, 2000–2015. *Arthritis & Rheumatology*, *70*(8), 1251–1255. https://doi.org/10.1002/art.40512

Interpretation of Fetal Heart Rate and Uterine Patterns

Antay L. Waters

▶ INTRODUCTION

The National Institute of Child Health and Human Development (NICHD) provides the standardized terminology for interpretation of fetal heart rate (FHR) and uterine patterns, originally proposed in 1997 and updated in 2008 (Macones et al., 2008). Using a standardized approach to FHR interpretation allows for a structured, systematic approach to antepartum and intrapartum care. The greatest strength of FHR monitoring is its ability to predict the absence of ongoing fetal hypoxic neurologic injury with a high degree of reliability, with the overarching goal of preventing fetal acidemia while simultaneously minimizing unnecessary interventions.

▶ OBJECTIVES

- Understand the current NICHD standardized terminology for the interpretation of FHR and uterine patterns (Table 6.1).
- Analyze the implications of various FHR and uterine pattern abnormalities related to care of the pregnant patient and the fetus.
- Review appropriate antepartum and intrapartum surveillance of the FHR and uterine patterns.

▶ KEY TERMS

- **Acceleration:** Apparent abrupt increase above the baseline with time from onset to peak <30 seconds. The peak must be 15 beats above the baseline and last 15+ seconds but <2 minutes. In pregnancies <32 weeks' gestation, accelerations are characterized by a peak 10 beats above the baseline lasting 10+ seconds but <2 minutes
- **Baseline rate:** Approximate FHR reported in 5-beats per minute (bpm) increments during a 10-minute period. At least 2 minutes of identifiable FHR segment in a 10-minute period is required to determine the baseline rate; otherwise, the baseline rate is considered indeterminate
- **Early deceleration:** Apparent gradual decrease below the baseline with onset to nadir ≥30 seconds, with the nadir associated with the peak of a uterine contraction
- **Fetal bradycardia:** Baseline rate <110 bpm
- **Fetal tachycardia:** Baseline rate >160 bpm
- **Intermittent:** Occurs in <50% of contractions in any 20-minute period
- **Late deceleration:** Apparent gradual decrease below the baseline with onset to nadir ≥30 seconds, with the nadir occurring after the peak of a uterine contraction
- **Prolonged:** Occurs for ≥2 minutes but <10 minutes. A change lasting ≥10 minutes is considered a baseline change
- **Recurrent:** Occurs in ≥50% of contractions in any 20-minute period
- **Sinusoidal pattern:** Visually smooth, sine wavelike pattern with 3- to 5-minute cycle frequency that lasts ≥20 minutes
- **Variability:** Fluctuation in the baseline FHR that is irregular in amplitude and frequency and distinct from accelerations and decelerations. There is no distinction between short- and long-term variability. Short-term variability is also referred to as beat-to-beat variability
  - ● **Absent variability:** Undetectable fluctuation in the baseline rate
  - ● **Minimal variability:** Fluctuation in the baseline rate that is visually detectable but ≤5 bpm

Table 6.1 2008 National Institute of Child Health and Human Development Terminology
for FHR Characteristics

Term	Definition
Baseline rate	Approximate FHR reported in 5-bpm increments during a 10-minute period. At least 2 minutes of identifiable FHR segment in a 10-minute period is required to determine the baseline rate; otherwise, the baseline rate is considered indeterminate.
Bradycardia	Baseline rate <110 bpm.
Tachycardia	Baseline rate >160 bpm.
Baseline variability *–Absent variability* *–Minimal variability* *–Moderate variability* *–Marked variability*	Fluctuation in the baseline FHR that is irregular in amplitude and frequency and distinct from accelerations and decelerations. There is no distinction between short- and long-term variability. Short-term variability is also referred to as beat-to-beat variability. –Undetectable fluctuation in the baseline rate. –Fluctuation in the baseline rate that is visually detectable but ≤5 bpm. –Fluctuation in the baseline rate between 6 and 25 bpm. –Fluctuation in the baseline rate >25 bpm.
Accelerations	Abrupt increases in the baseline rate, dependent on gestational age. • ≥32 weeks EGA: At least 15 bpm rise lasting ≥15 seconds and <2 minutes from onset to return to baseline. • <32 weeks EGA: At least 10 bpm rise lasting ≥10 seconds and <2 minutes from onset to return to baseline.
Early deceleration	Gradual decrease of the FHR with return to baseline associated with a uterine contraction. Gradual is defined as ≥30 seconds from onset to nadir. Nadir occurs no later than the peak of the contraction. Visually apparent and typically symmetrical. Most of the time, the onset, nadir, and recovery coincide with the beginning, peak, and end of the contraction, respectively.
Late deceleration	Gradual decrease of the FHR with return to baseline associated with a uterine contraction. Gradual is defined as ≥30 seconds from onset to nadir. Nadir occurs after the peak of the contraction. Visually apparent and typically symmetrical. Most of the time, the onset, nadir, and recovery occur after the beginning, peak, and end of the contraction, respectively.
Variable deceleration	Abrupt decrease in FHR. Abrupt is defined as <30 seconds from onset to nadir that is at least 15 bpm below baseline, lasting ≥15 seconds but <2 minutes. May occur irrespective of contractions.
Prolonged	Occurs for ≥2 minutes but <10 minutes. A change lasting ≥10 minutes is considered a baseline change.
Recurrent	Occurs ≥50% of contractions in any 20-minute period.
Intermittent	Occurs <50% of contractions in any 20-minute period.
Sinusoidal pattern	Visually smooth, sine wavelike pattern with 3- to 5-minute cycle frequency that lasts ≥20 minutes.

EGA, estimated gestational age; FHR, fetal heart rate.

Source: U.S. Department of Health and Human Services, National Institutes of Health, National Institute of Child Health and Human Development, 2008.

- **Moderate variability:** Fluctuation in the baseline rate between 6 and 25 bpm
- **Marked variability:** Fluctuation in the baseline rate >25 bpm
- **Variable deceleration:** Abrupt decrease ≥15 seconds, with onset to nadir <30 seconds

▶ CLASSIFICATION SYSTEMS OF ELECTRONIC FETAL HEART RATE AND UTERINE PATTERNS

The 2008 NICHD guidelines provide the current framework and definitions related to the interpretation of electronic FHR monitoring. First introduced in 1997 and updated in 2008, the NICHD guidelines have since been adopted by the American College of Obstetricians and Gynecologists (ACOG), the Society for Maternal-Fetal Medicine (SMFM), and the Association of Women's Health, Obstetric, and Neonatal Nurses (AWHONN).

DEFINITIONS

FHR characteristic definitions are presented in this chapter's key terms. All clinicians should be familiar with these definitions and use them consistently when discussing electronic FHR monitoring in clinical practice.

CHALLENGES RELATED TO THE INTERPRETATION OF ELECTRONIC FETAL HEART RATE MONITORING

Multiple challenges exist related to interpretation of electronic FHR monitoring, with the greatest challenge being inconsistency in definitions and thresholds for fetal acidemia, despite attempts by the NICHD to standardize. Clinically significant fetal acidemia is associated with an arterial umbilical cord pH <7.10 with a base excess less than −12 mmol/L (ACOG & AAP, 2014; Andres et al., 1999; Low et al., 1997).

Continuous electronic fetal monitoring (EFM) was developed in the 1960 s to assist in the diagnosis of fetal hypoxia during labor. Continuous EFM has been shown to reduce the incidence of neonatal seizures, but there been no beneficial effect in decreasing cerebral palsy or neonatal mortality. Poor interobserver and intraobserver reliability and significant variabilities may play a major role in its interpretation (Blackwell et al., 2019).

▶ SYSTEMATIC APPROACH TO ASSESSMENT OF FETAL HEART RATE AND UTERINE PATTERNS

Like most areas of medicine, evidence-based screening techniques and assessment methods are used to describe FHR and uterine patterns. The interpretation of FHR patterns has the unique position of subjectivity, primarily given the nature of visual interpretation and varying degrees of experience for those completing interpretation. In an attempt to improve interrater reliability, a systematic approach should be taken in the assessment of FHR and uterine patterns. Implementation of a systematic approach also assists the learner to develop skill and confidence in evaluation of fetal tracings.

1. **Baseline rate:** Is the rate within normal range, tachycardic, bradycardic, or indeterminate?
2. **Variability:** Is the variability absent, minimal, moderate, or marked?
3. **Accelerations and decelerations:** Are accelerations present? Are decelerations present? If decelerations are present, are they early, late, variable, or prolonged?
4. **Unusual characteristics:** Are any other unusual characteristics present, such as sinusoidal or pseudosinusoidal pattern? Evidence of fetal arrhythmia?
5. **Uterine activity:** What is the frequency, duration, and intensity of contractions? Resting tone?
6. **Changes over time:** How has the tracing changed over time?
7. **Tracing in comparison with clinical picture:** Does the tracing fit with the overall clinical picture? How does the clinical picture guide interpretation? Are there specific situations the team should prepare for? What potential complications should the team be aware of? Who needs to be aware of the current maternal-fetal status? What is the time frame for reevaluation? (Lydon & O'Brien-Abel, 2021)

▶ FETAL HEART RATE AND UTERINE ACTIVITY CHARACTERISTICS

BASELINE FETAL HEART RATE

The normal fetus maintains an overall consistent heart rate (HR) at rest, similar to an adult. While periods of excitement or stimulation lead to an increase in FHR, the FHR returns to its baseline once the stimulus is removed. As discussed in Chapter 3, the FHR is controlled through complex intertwined mechanisms including the fetal central nervous system (CNS), automatic nervous system, baroreceptors, chemoreceptors, and endocrine system. Normal beat-to-beat variation exists, appearing as a degree of fluctuation on the fetal monitoring strip.

The FHR baseline is the first characteristic evaluated, as it is the basis by which all other parameters are evaluated. According to the 2008 NICHD guidelines, the baseline FHR is the average FHR during any 10-minute segment rounded to an increment of 5 beats per minute and excludes accelerations, decelerations, and periods of marked variability. During this 10-minute segment, a minimum 2-minute segment that is not necessarily continuous must exist in order to determine the baseline. If this does not exist, the baseline is indeterminate. Normal FHR baselines range from 110 to 160 beats per minute.

Clinical Pearl

Proper baseline determination keeps you from missing other important FHR characteristics that may affect interpretation and patient management.

Tachycardia

Fetal tachycardia is classified as a baseline FHR >160 beats per minute (Figure 6.1). It represents an increase in sympathetic and/or decrease in parasympathetic fetal autonomic response and may be associated with a loss of variability (Freeman et al., 2012). In the presence of moderate variability, fetal tachycardia is not a sign of fetal distress (ACOG, 2010; Freeman et al., 2012; Parer, 1997). Fetal tachycardia may be either maternal or fetal in origin. Common causes of maternal tachycardia leading to fetal tachycardia include fever/maternal infection, maternal thyroid disorders, anxiety, dehydration, and medications such as beta sympathomimetics and phenothiazines. Fetal tachycardia may also result from hypoxia or acidosis, chorioamnionitis, or tachydysrhythmias. Correction of the underlying cause of maternal tachycardia typically brings the FHR back to a normal baseline. If fetal tachycardia is sustained for more than 50% of the tracing, it is considered sustained versus intermittent when periods of tachycardia alternate with a normal baseline. Sustained fetal tachycardia may tax fetal reserves due to increased myocardial oxygen demand. If associated with loss of variability and recurrent decelerations, consider potential fetal hypoxia (Nageotte, 2019).

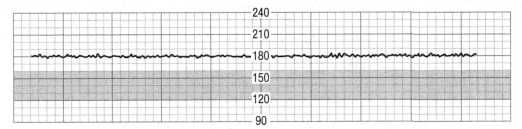

Figure 6.1 Fetal tachycardia.

Potential causes for sustained fetal tachycardia include maternal fever, infection, dehydration, certain medications (terbutaline, atropine, cocaine, and stimulants), medical conditions such as hypothyroidism, obstetric complications such as placental abruption, fetal bleeding, fetal anemia, fetal heart failure, fetal cardiac arrhythmias, fetal hypoxia, and/or metabolic acidemia (ACOG, 2010; Freeman et al., 2012; Miller, 2018). The primary provider should be notified and an attempt should be made to differentiate sinus tachycardia (ST) from supraventricular tachycardia (SVT). Fetal tachycardia associated with loss of variability or recurrent decelerations necessitates prompt, in-person evaluation by a provider. In the preterm fetus, consideration should be given to prompt evaluation in the setting of tachycardia, as the preterm fetus may develop hypoxia more rapidly secondary to their immunity and inability to compensate (Freeman et al., 2012).

Clinical Pearl

A rising FHR baseline requires investigation, as it could be one of the first signs of impending fetal hypoxia or acidosis.

Bradycardia

When the baseline FHR is <110 beats per minute for at least 10 minutes, fetal bradycardia is noted (Figure 6.2). A baseline FHR of 100 to 119 beats per minute in the absence of other nonreassuring patterns is not usually a sign of compromise. Fetal bradycardia may occur in a variety of acute or chronic conditions that may or may not lead to fetal hypoxia. In some cases, an FHR baseline between 80 and 110 beats per minute in conjunction with other reassuring signs such as moderate variability and/or accelerations may be accepted as normal for a particular fetus and consistent with an oxygenated, nonacidemic fetus. When the FHR falls below 60 beats per minute, fetal cardiac output is substantially decreased and may be associated with neonatal metabolic acidemia (Nageotte, 2019). A persistent baseline of 50 to 70 beats per minute may indicate a complete heart block not associated with fetal hypoxia. To confirm fetal bradycardia, simultaneous assessment of maternal HR is required. Bedside ultrasound may be required to confirm a bradycardic FHR.

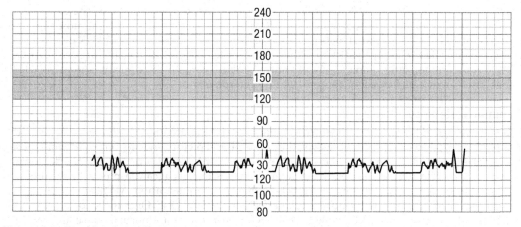

Figure 6.2 Fetal bradycardia.

Fetal bradycardia secondary to a hypoxic etiology will typically also exhibit variable and/or late decelerations secondary to decreased blood flow through either the placenta or the umbilical cord. As the fetus becomes increasingly hypoxic, carbon dioxide accumulates, leading to stimulation of chemoreceptors and compensatory increase in the FHR. If the increased FHR persists, baseline variability will decrease, and any periodic or episodic changes become more difficult to discern. The final phase culminates with terminal fetal bradycardia resulting from prolonged fetal hypoxia or asphyxia. Because of advances in fetal monitoring, this chain of events rarely ends in terminal bradycardia, as surgical intervention typically preempts its completion. Examples of hypoxic events related to fetal bradycardia include umbilical cord prolapse, maternal hypotension, excessive uterine stimulation, placental abruption, or uterine rupture. Sudden-onset fetal bradycardia is a medical emergency likely resulting from an acute change in maternal oxygenation, acute uteroplacental insufficiency, tachysystole, prolonged umbilical cord compression/occlusion, uterine rupture or placental abruption, or significant vagal stimulation (Parer, 1997).

Clinical Pearl

Remember that umbilical cord prolapse may be overt, funic (cord presentation), or occult.

Nonhypoxic causes of fetal bradycardia, such as vagal stimulation during the second stage of labor, is typically recoverable. During the second stage of labor, intense intracranial pressure occurs as the fetus descends through the maternal pelvis and vagina. Second-stage bradycardia may be seen in an adequately oxygenated fetus secondary to a normal vagal response. The key is recognizing the difference between hypoxic and nonhypoxic fetal bradycardia, done primarily through evaluation of baseline variability. A fetus with hypoxic bradycardia will have minimal to absent variability, while a fetus with nonhypoxic bradycardia will typically maintain moderate variability.

BASELINE FETAL HEART RATE VARIABILITY

Normal beat-to-beat variation of the FHR is physiologic. When evaluated in conjunction with the baseline as part of fetal monitoring interpretation, these visually apparent changes are referred to as variability. Variability can only be assessed during the same time period as baseline determination, as variability is a component of the baseline. There is no distinction between short-term (or beat-to-beat) variability and long-term variability.

Moderate Variability

Moderate variability (Figure 6.3) presents the most reassuring picture of fetal well-being and indicates that the fetal autonomic and CNS are well developed and well oxygenated. Moderate variability is defined as fluctuation in the FHR baseline from 6 to 25 beats per minute. It is one of the most important aspects of the FHR tracing related to its predictive features. Even in the setting of FHR decelerations, moderate variability is highly predictive of the absence of significant fetal metabolic acidosis (ACOG, 2010; Freeman et al., 2012; Parer, 1997). As such, careful attention to correctly determining FHR variability is an essential aspect of appropriate FHR interpretation.

Minimal Variability

When decreased FHR variability is noted (Figure 6.4), special attention should be paid given the risk for fetal hypoxia or acidosis. However, the entire clinical picture and any other potential causes for decreased variability must be considered prior to acting, such as maternal CNS depressant administration, fetal sleep cycles, fetal congenital anomalies, fetal tachycardia, preexisting neurologic abnormalities, prematurity, and maternal betamethasone administration. Medications that affect the maternal CNS are likely to produce similar effects on the fetal CNS. Once the medication is fully metabolized, variability should increase. While fetal sleep cycles are normal, these are transient periods that should alternate with periods of moderate variability approximately every 30 minutes. Consider that a fetus at <32 weeks' gestation may not have a fully developed autonomic nervous

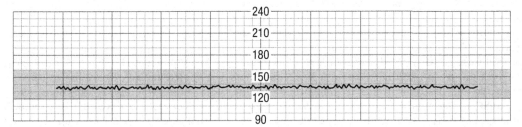

Figure 6.3 Moderate FHR variability.

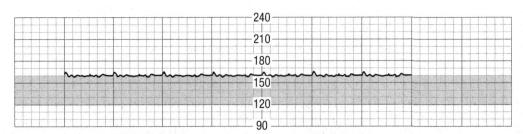

Figure 6.4 Minimal FHR variability.

system and therefore may have less variability. Despite this, once a fetus has established a certain level of variability, it has set a standard that should be maintained regardless of gestational age.

The overall correlation between acidemia and minimal or absent FHR variability is only approximately 23% (Parer et al., 2006). The primary cause of decreased FHR variability is fetal hypoxia. Loss of FHR variability secondary to hypoxia is related to diminished blood flow across the placenta and/or through the umbilical cord. Any condition or event resulting in diminished placental blood flow creates an opportunity for inadequate fetal oxygenation. If the hypoxia is significant enough to cause tissue hypoxia and metabolic acidosis, a loss of FHR variability may occur (Parer et al., 2006).

Absent Variability

Variability is considered absent (Figure 6.5) when it is no longer discernable on EFM. Decreased or absent variability should generally be confirmed by fetal scalp electrode monitoring when possible. Potential hypoxic causes of minimal to absent variability include cord prolapse/compression, maternal hypotension, tachysystole, placenta abruption, fetal tachycardia, and fetal dysrhythmia. Nonhypoxic causes include prematurity, fetal sleep cycle, fetal tachycardia, fetal anomaly (particularly cardiac and CNS related), maternal medication administration, and fetal dysrhythmia. The combination of late or severe variable decelerations with loss of variability is particularly ominous. Persistently minimal or absent FHR variability appears to be the most significant intrapartum sign of fetal compromise (Williams & Galerneau, 2003). It is imperative to observe for additional nonreassuring signs, including rising or falling baseline. However, the presence of good FHR variability may not always be predictive of a good outcome.

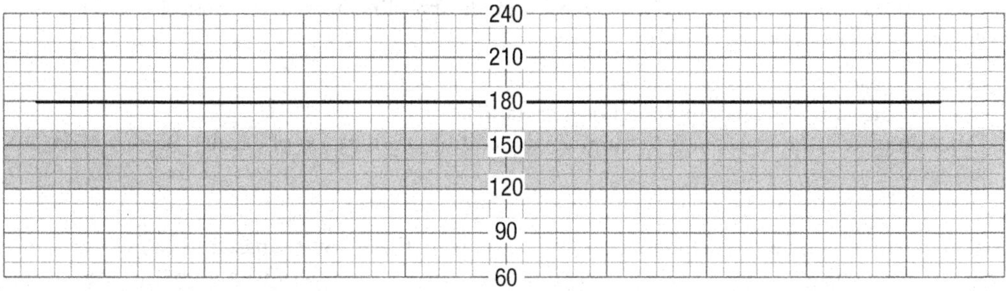

Figure 6.5 Absent FHR variability.

Marked Variability

While sometimes associated with fetal activity or stimulation, marked variability (Figure 6.6) may also be a sign that a fetus is hemodynamically compromised or mildly hypoxic (Parer, 1997). Potential

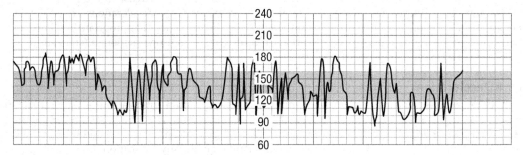

Figure 6.6 Marked FHR variability.

hypoxic causes for marked variability include umbilical cord prolapse/significant compression, maternal hypotension, tachysystole, and placental abruption. Emphasis should be placed on rapid causal determination and appropriate intervention through improving uteroplacental blood flow and perfusion.

Clinical Pearl

Variability can only be properly assessed when the baseline can be accessed.

ACCELERATIONS

FHR accelerations are transient increases in the FHR associated with fetal CNS stimulation and periods of increased fetal motor function. The absence of accelerations for more than 80 minutes correlates with increased neonatal morbidity (Patrick et al., 1984). Fetal scalp stimulation can be used to induce accelerations. There is about a 50% chance of acidosis in the fetus who fails to respond to stimulation in the presence of a nonreassuring pattern (Smith et al., 1986). This technique should not be used to verify the absence of acidemia during a deceleration of the FHR since there is insufficient literature to support its use during a deceleration.

DECELERATIONS

Decelerations are noted as transient decreases in the baseline related to periods of fetal stress. Decelerations are categorized based on:

1. Depth (measured in beats per minute)
2. Descent (measured in seconds from onset to nadir)
3. Duration (measured in seconds to minutes, depending on duration of deceleration from onset to recovery)
4. Timing (discussed in relation to contractions)

Other characterizing factors include shape and frequency; these are discussed in more detail in the following. Deepening of decelerations over time associated with absent to minimal variability may serve as an indicator of the need for intervention (Parer et al., 2006).

Early Decelerations

Early decelerations (Figure 6.7) are benign and uniform in shape. They begin near the onset of a uterine contraction, and the nadir occurs no later than the peak of the contraction. Early decelerations are caused by fetal head compression during a uterine contraction. As the uterine muscles become tighter and shorter, causing the uterus to decrease in size, space becomes even more limited for the fetus. This can occur in the few weeks before labor when there is less room for fetal movement and repositioning, as well as during labor. Early decelerations are often seen near the time of delivery. The pressure applied to the fetus during a uterine contraction may bend the fetal neck, causing vagal stimulation. Stimulation of the fetal vagus nerve may cause a decrease in the FHR seen as a deceleration that disappears immediately after the contraction. These decelerations are completely benign as they do not affect fetal oxygenation. Collectively, the presence of appropriate baseline FHR, variability, accelerations, and early decelerations indicates the reassuring function of fetal neurologic, autonomic, and cardiovascular systems.

Late Decelerations

Late decelerations (Figure 6.8) are also uniform in shape with a gradual onset and return to baseline. As opposed to early decelerations, late decelerations often begin just after a contraction, with their lowest point occurring after the nadir. These decelerations are associated with maternal and fetal conditions related to uteroplacental insufficiency. Any condition that predisposes

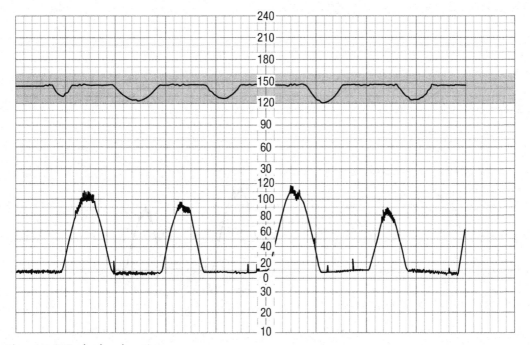

Figure 6.7 Early deceleration.

decreased uteroplacental blood flow may cause late decelerations. Some triggering circumstances include maternal hypotension secondary to epidural analgesia, maternal dehydration, significant maternal anemia, tachysystole, placental abruption, and fetal hypoxia. Other etiologies of late decelerations include maternal hypoxia, maternal hypertensive disorders, and fetal growth restriction.

Late decelerations associated with preserved beat-to-beat variability are typically mediated by arterial chemoreceptors in mild transient fetal hypoxia. When the level of oxygen in the fetal blood is below a partial pressure of oxygen (pO_2) of 15 to 20 mmHg, chemoreceptors are triggered, causing reflex alpha-adrenergic stimulation that constricts blood vessels in nonvital peripheral areas, such as the arms and legs, to divert more blood flow to vital organs, such as the heart and brain. Constriction of peripheral blood vessels leads to hypertension. The hypertension stimulates a baroreceptor-mediated vagal response that slows the HR. As this sequence only begins when fetal oxygenation is sufficiently reduced and occurs in a stepwise fashion, the onset of the FHR deceleration occurs after the onset of the uterine contraction, the deceleration occurs gradually, and the nadir of the deceleration is delayed from the peak of the contraction.

Late decelerations associated with absent variability not associated with maternal medication administration are cause for significant concern. If fetal hypoxia continues, the peripheral tissues cannot completely break down glucose and instead convert it to lactic acid. Acidemia may suppress the fetal nervous system, which becomes evident as decreased variability. As acidosis develops, the brainstem reflexes become blunted, and direct myocardial depression causes shallow decelerations. If myocardial depression is severe enough, late decelerations may be completely absent.

Variable Decelerations

Variable decelerations (Figure 6.9) are the most common type of fetal deceleration, typically occurring during the first and second stages of labor; however, they may also be present and noted during routine antepartum monitoring. Variable decelerations vary in shape, duration, and intensity. They often resemble the letters "U," "V," or "W" and may not have a constant relationship with uterine contractions. Lastly, variable decelerations are caused by compression of the umbilical cord, specifically the umbilical artery. Pressure on the cord initially occludes the umbilical vein, which results

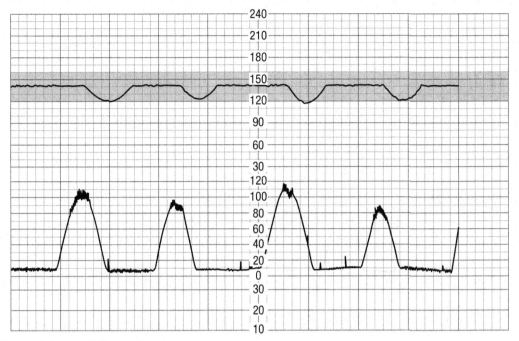

Figure 6.8 Late FHR deceleration.

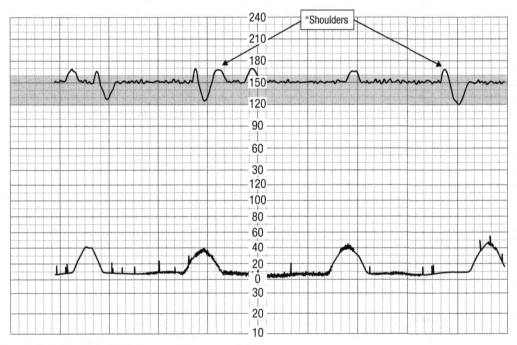

Figure 6.9 Variable FHR deceleration.

in an acceleration and indicates a healthy response. This is followed by occlusion of the umbilical artery, which results in a sharp deceleration as the result of arterial occlusion, decreased oxygenation, peripheral vasoconstriction, and comparatively abrupt reflex bradycardia. Oligohydramnios is associated with more frequent variable decelerations as the amniotic fluid has a protective role on the fetal umbilical cord. Variable decelerations usually indicate an obstruction to the fetal blood flow through the umbilical cord or compression of the umbilical vessels within the cord. If the decelerations are repetitive, the blood delivered to the fetus is significantly decreased, leading to fetal hypoxia and acidosis.

Variable decelerations may be vagally mediated through chemoreceptors or baroreceptors. "Shoulders" before or after a variable deceleration (see Figure 6.9) are thought to be caused by partial cord occlusion. This may occur before or after a variable deceleration. Assuming there is moderate variability associated with these decelerations, the overall pattern may be considered reassuring. Decreased venous return causes a baroreceptor-mediated acceleration. Hypertension and decreased arterial oxygen tension secondary to complete cord occlusion result in deceleration.

Prolonged Deceleration Versus Baseline Change

Prolonged decelerations are the most easily recognizable, as they are characterized by their duration. Prolonged decelerations range in length from 2 to 10 minutes and must have a ≥15 bpm decrease from baseline. These decelerations are measured from the time the FHR changes from the baseline through the return to baseline. While the etiology of a prolonged deceleration is varied, it is most often related to an acute event that causes transient interruption of maternal-fetal perfusion, including cord compression, tachysystole, or maternal hypotension. Prolonged decelerations may include an abrupt or gradual change in the FHR, may occur in response to fetal stress or changes in maternal hemodynamic status, and may occur as a single occurrence or repetitively. If a deceleration lasts for 10 minutes or more, it is characterized as a baseline change.

Quantification of Decelerations

FHR decelerations are quantified as either episodic or periodic. Episodic decelerations are not associated with uterine contractions. Periodic decelerations are associated with uterine contractions and include both early and late decelerations. Variable decelerations may be either episodic or periodic. Decelerations are considered recurrent if they occur in ≥50% of contractions in any 20-minute period, while intermittent decelerations occur in <50% of contractions in any 20-minute period.

Sinusoidal Pattern

A sinusoidal pattern (Figure 6.10) has regular amplitude and frequency and is excluded in the definition of variability. A sinusoidal pattern has a smooth, undulating pattern, or sine-like pattern, lasting at least 10 minutes with a fixed period of three to five cycles per minute and an amplitude of 5 to 15 beats per minute. Short-term variability is usually absent. A baseline FHR cannot be determined if a true sinusoidal pattern is present. It may also be complicated by other nonreassuring elements, such as variable, late, or prolonged decelerations.

Possible etiologies of sinusoidal patterns include severe fetal anemia, fetal hypoxia, or maternal medical administration. Sinusoidal pattern associated with fetal anemia is most often secondary to Rh isoimmunization; however, it may also result in maternal trauma, placental abruption, placenta previa, or other maternal-fetal hemorrhage. If a sinusoidal pattern is noted, ultrasound should be considered to rule out fetal ascites and hydrops.

Severe fetal hypoxia resulting in a sinusoidal pattern is often the result of the effect of hypoxia on the fetal autonomic nervous system. When a sinusoidal pattern is the result of fetal hypoxia, prompt delivery is indicated, with the understanding that some neurologic damage may have already occurred.

The most common cause of a sinusoidal pattern is maternal narcotic administration. When narcotic administration is the identified cause, the pattern is referred to as pseudosinusoidal or sinusoidal appearing, as the FHR pattern does not have a pathologic cause. The most common medications associated with a pseudosinusoidal pattern are butorphanol (Stadol), morphine sulfate, and meperidine (Demerol). It may also be seen with various illicit drugs, particularly opium—commonly seen in the Middle East (Keikha et al., 2016). It is imperative to obtain a reassuring tracing prior to medication administration of any narcotic so that if a sinusoidal-appearing pattern occurs, it can be

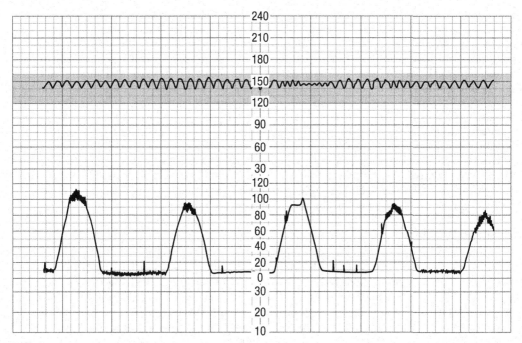

Figure 6.10 Sinusoidal FHR pattern.

determined that it was likely the result of recent medication administration and may be observed for resolution. Unlike a true sinusoidal pattern, pseudosinusoidal patterns have periods with a normal, reassuring tracing with a normal baseline and variability.

Fetal Arrhythmias

While fetal arrhythmias are diagnosed in approximately 1% to 3% of all pregnancies, malignant fetal dysrhythmias are relatively rare and occur in approximately 1 out of every 5,000 pregnancies (Yuan & Xu, 2020). The most lethal cardiac arrhythmias occur during otherwise normal pregnancies due to hidden depolarization and repolarization abnormalities and may be responsible for up to 10% of unexplained cases of fetal demise, unexplained hydrops, and prematurity (Crotti et al., 2013).

In most cases, fetal premature ventricular contractions (PVCs) and premature atrial contractions (PACs) do not require treatment and spontaneously resolve prior to delivery. In approximately 2% to 3% of cases, couplets are seen and increase the risk of SVT by approximately 10%. In cases with blocked atrial bigeminy (BAB), a low baseline range from 70 to 90 bpm may be seen. BAB is not associated with fetal hydrops, and no treatment is required. It is often misdiagnosed as a second-degree atrioventricular (AV) block, which is extremely rare, and should be followed by someone familiar with this type of arrhythmia to avoid management mistakes due to misidentification (Bravo-Valenzuela et al., 2018).

Fetal tachyarrhythmias may be classified as ST, SVT, or ventricular tachycardia (VT). SVT is the most common form of fetal tachycardia, occurring in 70% to 75% of all cases, and VT is the rarest (Krapp et al., 2003). ST is typically related to fetal distress secondary to hypoxia or a maternal condition such as thyroid storm, anemia, administration of β-agonists, and infections such as chorioamnionitis and cytomegalovirus (CMV). In these cases, no specific antiarrhythmic therapy is indicated, but rather the underlying cause should be identified and treated (Bravo-Valenzuela et al., 2018).

While persistent fetal bradycardia is rare, approximately 30% of all cases of sustained bradycardia are caused by BAB, resulting in a well-tolerated, lower-than-normal ventricular rate of 70 to 90 bpm. Typically, this spontaneously converts to sinus rhythm prior to delivery, and no treatment is required. Clinically insignificant episodes of fetal bradycardia frequently occur, particularly during the second trimester, resolve spontaneously within minutes, and are considered to be benign (Bravo-Valenzuela et al., 2018).

UTERINE ACTIVITY

Because FHR tracings are interpreted in relation to uterine activity (Figure 6.11), understanding how to describe uterine activity is imperative to appropriate fetal monitoring interpretation. Evaluation of uterine activity has four parts:

1. **Frequency:** Describes the time in minutes from the start of one contraction to the start of the next contraction.
2. **Duration:** Describes the length of the contraction in seconds. A tetanic contraction is any contraction that lasts longer than 2 minutes.
3. **Intensity:** Describes the strength of the contraction. May be assessed by palpation or intrauterine pressure catheter (IUPC).
   a. **Palpation:** Mild, moderate, and strong
   b. **IUPC:** Montevideo units (MVUs) or mmHg
4. **Resting tone:** Describes the tone of the uterus between contractions. May be assessed by palpation or IUPC.
   a. **Palpation:** Soft or firm
   b. **IUPC:** mmHg

During active labor, normal uterine activity consists of contractions every 2 to 3 minutes, lasting 80 to 90 seconds, that are strong to palpation. Uterine contractions are quantified as the number of contractions present in a 10-minute window, averaged over 30 minutes. Normal uterine activity includes five or fewer contractions in 10 minutes, averaged over a 30-minute window. Tachysystole, previously referred to as uterine hyperstimulation, is defined as more than five contractions in 10 minutes, averaged over a 30-minute window. Consideration must be given in both spontaneous and stimulated labor. Tachysystole should always be qualified as to the presence or absence of associated FHR decelerations. Coupling or tripling occurs when two or three contractions occur with little to no resting tone repeatedly in regular intervals. This may occur as a result of dysfunctional labor or when oxytocin receptors become saturated and downregulate as a result of excessive oxytocin exposure (Phaneuf et al., 2000).

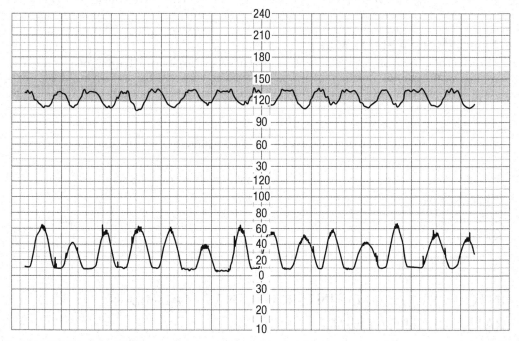

Figure 6.11 Uterine activity.

▶ INTERPRETATION OF ELECTRONIC FETAL HEART RATE MONITORING

Once you understand each of the components of FHR interpretation, the NICHD three-tier interpretation system should be applied.

CATEGORY I: NORMAL

Category I FHR tracings are strongly predictive of normal fetal acid-base status at the time of interpretation. In order to be classified as category I, the FHR tracing must show *ALL* of the following:

1. Baseline FHR 110 to 160 bpm
2. Moderate variability
3. Accelerations: may be present or absent
4. Early decelerations: may be present
5. No late or variable decelerations

CATEGORY II: INDETERMINATE

Category II, or indeterminate, FHR tracings are not predictive of abnormal fetal acid-base status but do require increased surveillance. Category II tracings create a very broad classification that may include any of the following:

1. Fetal tachycardia
2. Fetal bradycardia without absent variability
3. Minimal variability
4. Absent variability without recurrent decelerations
5. Marked variability
6. Absence of accelerations after stimulation
7. Recurrent variable decelerations with minimal or moderate variability
8. Prolonged deceleration ≥2 minutes but <10 minutes
9. Recurrent late decelerations with moderate variability
10. Variable decelerations with other characteristics such as slow return to baseline

CATEGORY III: ABNORMAL

Category III FHR tracings are predictive of abnormal fetal-acid base status at the time of interpretation. Depending on the clinical situation, efforts to expeditiously resolve the underlying cause of the abnormal FHR pattern should be made. The FHR tracing is considered category III if *EITHER* of the following are present:

1. Sinusoidal pattern
2. Absent variability with recurrent late or variable decelerations or fetal bradycardia

---

Clinical Pearl

Any fetal monitoring strip that is not explicitly category I or category III is classified as category II and requires additional evaluation.

▶ INTERPRETATION OF INTERMITTENT FETAL HEART RATE AUSCULTATION

Intermittent FHR auscultation presents a different set of challenges, as there is likely to be even greater discrepancy in both interobserver and intraobserver reliability; however, the three-tiered system still has implication and use during intermittent auscultation. During intermittent auscultation, only two tiers are used and are consistent with the NICHD system. When using intermittent auscultation to determine baseline, the FHR should be counted for at least 15 to 30 seconds after a contraction to detect for periodic changes. This allows for assessment for the presence of changes in the FHR as well as allows for characterization of changes, such as abrupt versus gradual (Wisner & Holschuh, 2018).

Category I FHR characteristics by auscultation include *ALL* of the following:

1. Normal FHR baseline between 110 and 160 bpm
2. Regular rhythm
3. Presence or absence of accelerations
4. Absence of decelerations

Category II FHR characteristics by auscultation include *ANY* of the following:

1. Irregular rhythm
2. Presence of decelerations
3. Fetal tachycardia
4. Fetal bradycardia

Category I FHR characteristics are reassuring and predictive of fetal well-being at the time they are obtained. Category II FHR characteristics cannot be classified as normal or abnormal without obtaining information related to variability; they require additional evaluation, possibly including a period of continuous fetal monitoring to confirm reassuring FHR characteristics (Lydon et al., 2009).

Clinical Pearl

The positive predictive value of intrapartum fetal monitoring in predicting cerebral palsy is virtually zero, while the negative predictive value is nearly 100%.

▶ KEY POINTS

■ Use of the standardized terminology developed by the NICHD to describe and interpret EFM can help reduce miscommunication among healthcare providers.

■ Late and variable decelerations both potentially indicate a predisposition to hypoxic injury and/or acidosis of the fetus and should prompt further investigation, closer observation, and possible intervention on the part of the obstetric clinician.

■ NICHD standardized terminology still applies with slight modification during intermittent auscultation.

■ Variability is the single greatest predictor of fetal oxygenation status.

CASE STUDY

April is a 37-year-old G3P0111 patient at 34 weeks and 2 days' gestation presenting to OB triage for evaluation of contractions every 5 minutes for the last 6 hours. Her initial cervical exam was 2/50/-3 with bulging membranes. After an hour of category I tracing, she complains of sudden-onset leaking of clear fluid. Repeat cervical exam is 4/90/-2. April is admitted to labor and delivery for preterm premature rupture of membranes (PPROM) and management of active preterm labor. Cephalic presentation is confirmed via bedside ultrasound. Internal monitors are placed and amnioinfusion initiated after a period of recurrent variable decelerations. Following this event, April's tracing changes, as seen in the following.

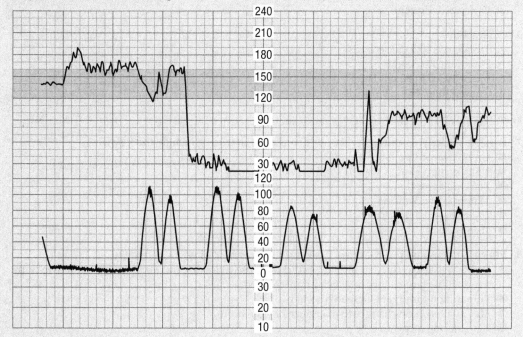

Answer the following, and then see in the "Case Study Answers" for correct answers.

1. Baseline FHR: _____

2. Variability: _____

3. Accelerations: Present or absent? _____

4. Decelerations:
    a. Early: Present or absent? _____
    b. Variable: Present or absent? _____
    c. Late: Present or absent? _____
    d. Prolonged: Present or absent? _____

5. Contractions:
    a. Frequency: _____
    b. Duration: _____
    c. Intensity: _____
    d. Resting tone: _____

6. Interpretation: Category _____

7. Discuss possible underlying causes for the sudden change in tracing, including rationale.

8. Determine priority actions and interventions based on the current tracing.

(See answers next page.)

CASE STUDY ANSWERS

1. Baseline FHR: Indeterminate

2. Variability: Indeterminate

3. Accelerations: Present

4. Decelerations:
   a. Early: Absent
   b. Variable: Absent
   c. Late: Absent
   d. Prolonged: Present

5. Contractions:
   a. Frequency: 30 to 50 seconds
   b. Duration: 30 seconds
   c. Intensity: 60 to 80 mmHg
   d. Resting tone: 15 to 20 mmHg

6. Interpretation: Category II

7. Possible underlying causes for the sudden change in tracing include the following:
   - Umbilical cord prolapse
   - Uterine rupture
   - Placenta abruption
   - Maternal hypotension
   - Uteroplacental insufficiency
   - Tachysystole

8. Priority actions and interventions based on the current tracing are as follows:
   - Cervical exam to rule out umbilical cord prolapse following initiation of amnioinfusion with manual displacement of fetal head if discovered
   - Preparation for urgent Cesarean section
   - Maternal position changes to maximize oxygenation
   - Considering tocolysis

KNOWLEDGE CHECK: CHAPTER 6

1. When comparing early and late decelerations, a distinguishing factor is:
   A) Onset time to baseline return
   B) Onset time to nadir
   C) Timing in relation to contractions

2. The underlying cause of early decelerations is:
   A) Decreased baroreceptor response
   B) Increased stroke volume (SV)
   C) Increased vagal response

3. Following an ultrasound consistent with a decreased amniotic fluid index, a term patient is admitted in early labor. The resulting fetal heart rate (FHR) decelerations:
   A) Are not necessarily associated with contractions
   B) Occur after the peak of the contraction
   C) Occur prior to the peak of the contraction

4. Fetal hypoxia is best described as decreased oxygen in the:
   A) Amniotic fluid
   B) Blood
   C) Tissue

5. Stimulation of the fetal parasympathetic nervous system causes the fetal heart rate (FHR) to:
   A) Decrease
   B) Increase
   C) Remain the same

6. Activation of the fetal peripheral chemoreceptors results in the fetal heart rate (FHR):
   A) Decreasing
   B) Increasing
   C) Remaining the same

7. A common medication-related cause of sinusoidal-appearing tracing is:
   A) Betamethasone
   B) Butorphanol
   C) Terbutaline

(See answers next page.)

1. C) Timing in relation to contractions

Early and late decelerations are distinguished based on the relationship of the nadir to the contraction. Onset time to nadir is used in differentiating variable decelerations, as they are abrupt. Return to baseline may be used to determine if a deceleration is prolonged or not.

2. C) Increased vagal response

Early decelerations are the result of a vagal response secondary to the compression of the fetal head. Increased baroreceptor response causes a decrease in fetal heart rate (FHR). Because the fetal heart operates near its peak, SV does not change significantly.

3. A) Are not necessarily associated with contractions

Variable decelerations are seen in the setting of oligohydramnios related to the increased risk of cord compression due to lack of adequate amniotic fluid. As early decelerations are associated with fetal head compression and late decelerations are seen in uteroplacental insufficiency, they are not a risk inherent primarily to oligohydramnios.

4. C) Tissue

Fetal hypoxia occurs due to an inadequate supply of oxygen on the cellular level that leads to metabolic acidosis. Decreased oxygen in the blood is known as fetal hypoxemia. Amniotic fluid does not carry oxygen.

5. A) Decrease

Stimulation of the fetal parasympathetic nervous system causes the FHR to decrease. Stimulation of the fetal sympathetic nervous system is responsible for increases in FHR.

6. A) Decreasing

Activation of peripheral chemoreceptors results in a decrease in the FHR, most often late and variable decelerations. The sympathetic nervous system is responsible for increases in FHR.

7. B) Butorphanol

Narcotics may cause a pseudosinusoidal pattern that spontaneously resolves when the medication effect wears off. Betamethasone may cause a decrease in variability. Terbutaline may cause an increase in baseline rate.

8. Which of the following is most likely responsible for the following tracing?

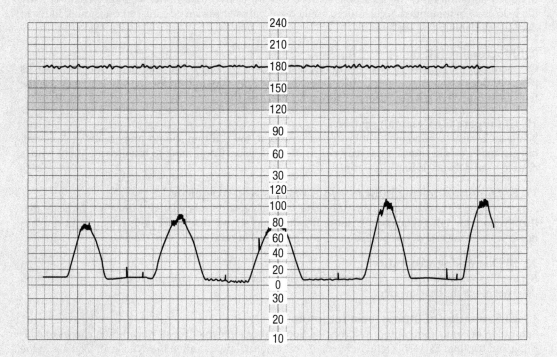

   A) Maternal betamethasone administration
   B) Maternal dehydration
   C) Maternal hypotension

9. The fetus compensates for decreased maternal circulating volume by increasing cardiac output (CO) by:
   A) Decreasing heart rate (HR)
   B) Increasing HR
   C) Increasing stroke volume (SV)

10. During monitoring of a dichorionic/diamniotic twin gestation in labor, Twin B has a prolonged deceleration for 8 minutes. The last cervical exam was 3/50/-3. What should the next action be?
    A) Apply oxygen
    B) Continue to monitor
    C) Prepare for Cesarean section

11. When providing patient education related to electronic fetal monitoring (EFM), the most appropriate statement is:
    A) "A normal tracing indicates that your baby is healthy."
    B) "A normal tracing indicates your baby is well-oxygenated."
    C) "Continuous fetal monitoring will ensure a better outcome for your baby."

12. Betamethasone given to the pregnant patient can transiently affect the fetal heart rate (FHR) by:
    A) Changing baseline rate
    B) Decreasing variability
    C) Increasing variability

13. Which of the following is the most likely cause of coupling?
    A) Excessive fetal movement
    B) Late decelerations
    C) Saturation of oxytocin receptors

(See answers next page.)

8. B) Maternal dehydration

Maternal dehydration is the most likely cause of fetal tachycardia. Maternal hypotension is more likely to cause a prolonged deceleration, while maternal magnesium administration is more likely to decrease variability and the baseline.

9. B) Increasing HR

CO increases in response to changes in HR or SV (CO = HR × SV). The fetal heart operates near its peak; SV does not change significantly. Therefore, the only way to increase the CO is to increase the fetal heart rate (FHR). A decrease in FHR would decrease CO.

10. C) Prepare for Cesarean section

While a Cesarean section may not be urgently needed, the clinician should prepare for it. Applying oxygen may be done; however, it may not resolve the issue. Continuing to monitor a patient who is remote from delivery is not appropriate.

11. B) "A normal tracing indicates your baby is well-oxygenated."

A normal tracing is consistent with adequate fetal oxygenation; however, it does not indicate that there is no underlying fetal complication. Research has shown that continuous fetal monitoring has not decreased the rate of cerebral palsy or ensured a better outcome.

12. B) Decreasing variability

Betamethasone is known to temporarily decrease, not increase, variability. Steroid administration does not affect the baseline rate.

13. C) Saturation of the oxytocin receptors

Saturation of oxytocin receptors and dysfunctional labor are two of the most common causes of coupling and tripling. Excessive fetal movement and maternal dehydration may cause an increase in the baseline but do not affect uterine activity.

14. When using intermittent auscultation to determine the baseline, the fetal heart rate (FHR) should be counted after a contraction for how many seconds?
    A) 10 to 15
    B) 15 to 30
    C) 30 to 60

15. Which of the following fetal heart rate (FHR) characteristics can be determined using intermittent auscultation?
    A) Baseline rate
    B) Type of deceleration
    C) Variability

16. What is the *most* probable cause of recurrent late decelerations?
    A) Cord compression
    B) Head compression
    C) Uteroplacental insufficiency

17. As a result of the intrinsic fetal response to oxygen deprivation, increased catecholamine levels cause the peripheral blood flow to decrease while the blood flow to vital organs increases. These flow changes along with increased catecholamine secretions have what effect on fetal blood pressure and fetal heart rate (FHR)?
    A) Increase blood pressure and decrease heart rate (HR)
    B) Increase blood pressure and increase HR
    C) Increase blood pressure with no change to HR

18. Regarding the reliability of electronic fetal monitoring (EFM) interpretation, there is:
    A) Good interobserver and intraobserver reliability
    B) Poor interobserver and intraobserver reliability
    C) Poor interobserver reliability and good intraobserver reliability

19. Which of the following is the *least likely* cause of the following tracing?

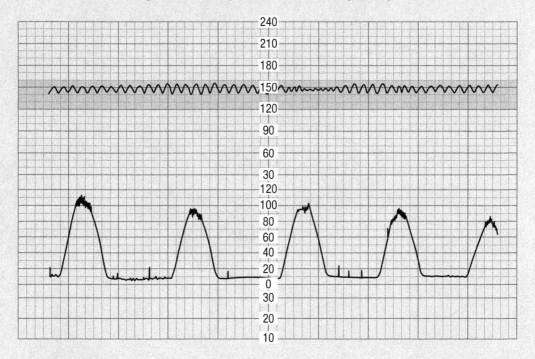

    A) Fetal anemia
    B) Maternal intracranial hemorrhage
    C) Ruptured vasa previa

(See answers next page.)

14. B) 15 to 30 seconds

When using intermittent auscultation to determine baseline, the FHR should be counted for at least 15 to 30 seconds after a contraction to detect for periodic changes. This allows assessment for the presence of changes in the FHR as well as allows for characterization of changes, such as abrupt versus gradual.

15 A) Baseline rate

Only a baseline rate and presence or absence of accelerations and decelerations may be determined by intermittent auscultation. Variability and type of deceleration can only be determined by evaluation of a continuous tracing.

16. C) Uteroplacental insufficiency

Late decelerations are most often caused by some form of uteroplacental insufficiency. Variable decelerations are most often caused by some form of interruption of blood flow through the umbilical cord, typically cord compression. Early decelerations result from compression of the fetal head.

17. A) Increase blood pressure and decrease heart rate (HR)

As a response to oxygen deprivation, the FHR will decrease and blood pressure will increase due to increased catecholamines.

18. B) Poor interobserver and intraobserver reliability

It is hypothesized that one of the reasons little impact has been made on cerebral palsy rates is secondary to poor interobserver and intraobserver reliability related to external fetal monitoring interpretation.

19. B) Maternal intracranial hemorrhage

Fetal anemia and ruptured vasa previa are both possible causes of a sinusoidal pattern. While a fetal intracranial hemorrhage is a potential cause of a sinusoidal pattern, a maternal intracranial hemorrhage is not.

20. A 37-year-old G1P000 patient at 38 weeks' gestation is being induced for oligohydramnios. The cervical exam is 5/80/-2 with intact amniotic membranes, and the patient has just received an epidural. Which of the following could result in the following fetal tracing?

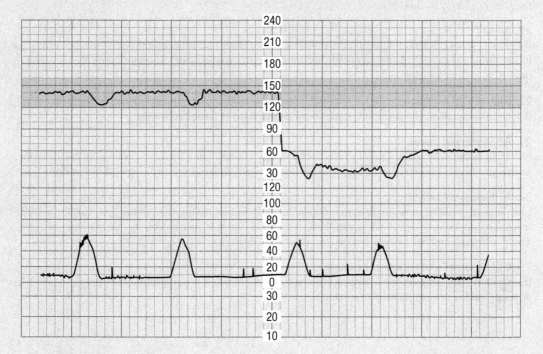

A) Maternal hypotension
B) Umbilical cord prolapse
C) Uterine rupture

21. The clinician is reviewing a nonstress test. 10×10 accelerations with moderate variability are noted. For which gestational age, in weeks, would this be considered a reactive fetal tracing?
A) 30
B) 32
C) 34

22. A tetanic contraction lasts longer than *at least* how many minutes?
A) 1
B) 2
C) 3

23. All of the following are likely causes of a prolonged deceleration *except:*
A) Maternal fever
B) Prolapsed cord
C) Tachysystole

24. Which part of the nervous system reduces the fetal heart rate (FHR) and maintains variability through stimulation of the vagus nerve?
A) Parasympathetic
B) Peripheral
C) Sympathetic

25. According to the American College of Obstetricians and Gynecologists (ACOG), intermittent auscultation is appropriate for:
A) All pregnancies
B) Complicated pregnancies
C) Uncomplicated pregnancies

(See answers next page.)

20. A) Maternal hypotension

A prolonged deceleration immediately after epidural placement is most likely secondary to maternal hypotension. While umbilical cord prolapse and uterine rupture may cause a prolonged deceleration, they are not likely in this situation.

21. A) 30

Prior to 32 weeks, a fetal tracing is considered reactive with 10×10 accelerations as long as the fetus has not previously had 15×15 accelerations noted. At 32+ weeks, 15×15 accelerations are required to qualify as an acceleration.

22. B) 2

A tetanic contraction is a contraction that lasts longer than at least 2 minutes.

23. A) Maternal fever

Maternal fever will likely lead to fetal tachycardia but will not cause a prolonged deceleration. Tachysystole and umbilical cord prolapse are both known causes for a prolonged deceleration.

24. A) Parasympathetic

The parasympathetic nervous system reduces the FHR and increases, then maintains, variability with increasing gestational age. The sympathetic nervous system is responsible for decreasing the FHR. The peripheral nervous system has no impact on the FHR.

25. C) Uncomplicated pregnancies

Intermittent auscultation is not appropriate for all pregnancies or for complicated pregnancies. It is appropriate for uncomplicated pregnancies.

▶ REFERENCES

American College of Obstetricians and Gynecologists. (2010). Practice bulletin 116: Management of intrapartum fetal heart rate tracings. *Obstetrics & Gynecology, 116*(5), 1232–1240.

American College of Obstetricians and Gynecologists & American Academy of Pediatrics. (2014). Neonatal encephalopathy and neurologic outcome. *Pediatrics, 133*(5), e1482–e1488. https://doi .org/10.1542/peds.2014-0724

Andres, R. L., Saade, G., Gilstrap, L. C., Wilkins, I., Witlin, A., Zlatnik, F., & Hankins, G. V. (1999). Association between umbilical blood gas parameters and neonatal morbidity and death in neonates with pathologic fetal anemia. *American Journal of Obstetrics & Gynecology, 181*(4), 867–871. https://doi.org/10.1016/s0002-9378(99)70316-9

Blackwell, S., Grobman, W., Antoniewicz, L., Hutchinson, M., & Bannerman, C. (2011). Interobserver and intraobserver reliability of the NICHD 3-tier fetal heart rate interpretation system. *American Jounral of Obstetrics and Gynecology, 205*(4), 378.31-378.e5. https://doi .org/10.1016/j.ajog.2011.06.086

Bravo-Valenzuela, N. J., Rocha, L. A., Machado Nardozza, L. M., & Araujo Júnior, E. (2018). Fetal cardiac arrhythmias: Current evidence. *Annals of Pediatric Cardiology, 11*(2), 148–163. https://doi.org/10.4103/apc.APC_134_17

Crotti, L., Tester, D. J., White, W. M., Bartos, D. C., Insolia, R., Besana, A., Kunic, J. D., Will, M. L., Velasco, E. J., Bair, J. J., Ghidoni, A., Cetin, I., Van Dyke, D. L., Wick, M. J., Brost, B., Delisle, B. P., Facchinetti, F., George, A. L., Schwartz, P. J., & Ackerman, M. J. (2013). Long QT syndrome-associated mutations in intrauterine fetal death. *Journal of the American Medical Association, 309*(14), 1473–1482. https://doi.org/10.1001/jama.2013.3219

Freeman, R. K., Garite, T. J., Nageotte, M. P., & Miller, L. A. (2012). *Fetal heart rate monitoring* (4th ed.). Lippincott Williams & Wilkins.

Keikha, F., Vahdani, F. G., & Latifi, S. (2016). The effects of maternal opium abuse on fetal heart rate using non-stress test. *Iran Journal of Medical Science, 41*(6), 479–485.

Krapp, M., Kohl, T., Simpson, J. M., Sharland, G. K., Katalinic, A., & Gembruch, U. (2003). Review of diagnosis, treatment, and outcome of fetal atrial flutter compared with supraventricular tachycardia. *Heart, 89*(8), 913–917. https://doi.org/10.1136/heart.89.8.913

Low, J. A., Victory, R., & Derrick, E. J. (1997). Threshold of metabolic acidosis for intrapartum fetal asphyxia with metabolic acidosis. *Obstetrics & Gynecology, 93*(2), 285–291. https://doi .org/10.1016/s0029-7844(98)00441-4

Lydon, A., & O'Brien-Abel, N. (2021). Fetal heart rate interpretation. In A. Lyndon, & K. Wisner (Eds.), *Fetal heart monitoring principles and practices* (6th ed., pp. 121–122). Kendall Hunt.

Lydon, A., O'Brien-Abel, N., & Simpson, K. R. (2009). Interpretation of fetal heart monitoring. In A. Lyndon, & L. U. Ali (Eds.), *Fetal heart monitoring principles and practices* (4th ed., vol. 99, pp. 101–133). Kendall Hunt.

Macones, G., Hankins, G., Spong, C., Hauth, J., & Moore, T. (2008). The 2008 National Institute of Child Health and Human Development workshop report on electronic fetal monitoring: Update on definitions, interpretation, and research guidelines. *Obstetrics & Gynecology, 112*(3), 661–666. https://doi.org/10.1097/AOG.0b013e3181841395

Miller, L. A. (2018). Uterine activity: What you don't know can hurt you. *The American Journal of Maternal Child Nursing, 43*(3), 180. https://doi.org/10.1097/NMC.0000000000000431

Nageotte, M. P. (2019). Intrapartum fetal surveillance. In R. Resnik, C. J. Lockwood, T. R. Moore, M. F. Freene, J. A. Copel, & R. M. Silver (Eds.), *Cresy & Resnik's maternal-fetal medicine: Principles and practices* (8th ed., pp. 564–582). Elsevier.

Parer, J. (1997). *Handbook of fetal heart rate monitoring* (2nd ed.). W. B. Saunders.

Parer, J. T., King, T., Flanders, S., Fox, M., & Kilpatrick, J. (2006). Fetal acidemia and electronic fetal heart rate patterns: Is there evidence of an association? *Journal of Maternal-Fetal & Neonatal Medicine, 19*(5), 289–294. https://doi.org/10.1080/14767050500526172

Patrick, J., Carmichael, L., Chess, L., & Staples, C. (1984). Accelerations of the human fetal heart rate at 38 to 40 weeks' gestational age. *American Journal of Obstetrics & Gynecology, 148*(1), 35–41. https://doi.org/10.1016/s0002-9378(84)80028-9

Phaneuf, S., Rodriguez Linares, B., TambyRaja, R. L., MacKenzie, I. Z., & Lopez Bernal, A. (2000). Loss of myometrial oxytocin receptors during oxytocin-induced and oxytocin-augmented labour. *Journal of Reproduction and Fertility, 120*(1), 91–97. https://doi.org/10.1530/jrf.0.1200091

Smith, C. V., Nguyen, H. N., Phelan, J. P., & Paul, R. H. (1986). Intrapartum assessment of fetal well-being: A comparison of fetal acoustic stimulation with acid-base determinations. *American Journal of Obstetrics & Gynecology, 155*(4), 726–728. https://doi.org/10.1016/s0002-9378(86)80007-2

Williams, K. P., & Galerneau, F. (2003). Intrapartum fetal heart rate patterns in the prediction of neonatal acidemia. *American Journal of Obstetrics & Gynecology, 188*(3), 820–823. https://doi.org/10.1067/mob.2003.183

Wisner, K., & Holschuh, C. (2018). Fetal heart rate auscultation, 3rd ed. *Nursing for Women's Health, 2*, e1–e32. https://doi.org/10.1016/j.nwh.2018.10.001

Yuan, S. M., & Xu, Z. Y. (2020). Fetal arrhythmias: Prenatal evaluation and intrauterine therapeutics. *Italian Journal of Pediatrics, 46*, 21. https://doi.org/10.1186/s13052-020-0785-9

Interventions for Fetal Heart Rate and Uterine Pattern Abnormalities

Antay L. Waters

▶ INTRODUCTION

Following interpretation of electronic fetal monitoring (EFM) strips, interventions are often required to correct noted abnormalities in order to maintain adequate fetal oxygenation. By developing a strong understanding of fetal physiology, clinicians have the ability to appropriately select and implement interventions to maximize fetal oxygenation and improve overall outcomes. Overall fetal well-being requires not only a well-oxygenated fetus but a well-oxygenated and hemodynamically stable pregnant patient. Understanding interventions for nonreassuring fetal status through intrauterine resuscitation techniques, avoiding and correcting maternal hypotension secondary to regional anesthesia, coaching modified maternal pushing efforts, understanding fetal arrhythmias, and avoiding and/or correcting uterine tachysystole allow the clinician to have an arsenal of options for supporting the well-oxygenated fetus.

▶ OBJECTIVES

- Analyze available interventions and determine appropriateness for given clinical scenarios.
- Relate fetal heart rate (FHR) and uterine pattern abnormalities to correctable causes while implementing appropriate interventions.
- Discuss shared decision-making with the perinatal team related to interventions based on FHR and uterine pattern abnormalities.

▶ KEY TERMS

- **Arrhythmia:** Any irregular heartbeat
- **Tocolysis:** Inhibition of uterine contractions through interventions
- **Uterotonic agents:** Medications that produce adequate uterine contractions

▶ INTERVENTIONS FOR CATEGORY II AND CATEGORY III FETAL HEART RATE PATTERNS

When interventions are indicated for category II and category III EFM, action should be taken within the recommended time frame of 60 minutes (Clark et al., 2013). While the vast majority of fetuses are well-oxygenated and nonacidotic, many will have a category II tracing at some point during either the antepartum or the intrapartum period. Based on limited data, various techniques and interventions may be used to improve category II tracings and overall fetal status. Category III tracings are rare, occurring in approximately .9% of fetuses within 30 minutes of delivery. Approximately 20% of pregnant patients will have one or more interventions related to category II tracings prior to delivery, with the majority of these occurring during the first stage of labor (Reddy et al., 2021). Shared decision-making should involve all members of the patient care team and the patient to ensure that the most appropriate intervention(s) are implemented.

INTRAUTERINE RESUSCITATION TECHNIQUES

Intrauterine resuscitation techniques include a variety of interventions given to the pregnant patient to improve fetal oxygenation by improving placental blood flow, increasing maternal blood oxygen concentration, or alleviating cord compression. Having a strong understanding of these interventions and their appropriate use increases the patient's chance of successful intervention and improvement in the EFM tracing. Evidence exists to support the use of various interventions, including maternal position changes, IV fluid administration, oxygen administration, amnioinfusion, and tocolytics; however, the available evidence is sometimes contradictory (Bullens et al., 2015). It is important for clinicians to remember to allow adequate time, at least 60 seconds, for the FHR to recover after changing positions before adding additional interventions or position changes.

Maternal Position Changes

While the left lateral position is ideal for improving and promoting fetal circulation, other positions may be necessary to improve overall fetal status depending on the clinical situation. Other positions for consideration include right lateral and knee-chest positions, which relieve pressure from the maternal inferior vena cava, allowing increased venous return and cardiac output. In turn, the increased venous return and increased cardiac output may improve uteroplacental perfusion in order to improve late decelerations. Maternal position changes also have the ability to improve variable decelerations by relieving cord compression (Raghurman, 2020).

Intravenous Fluid Administration

In cases where nonreassuring fetal tracings are attributed to fetal hypoxia related to poor placental perfusion, IV fluids may be administered in order to increase maternal intravascular volume, thereby improving placental perfusion and fetal oxygenation. In a 2005 randomized control trial comparing 500-mL versus 1-L IV fluid boluses, the 1-L bolus was associated with a significant increase in fetal oxygen saturation (Simpson & James, 2005). An added effect of IV fluid administration is tocolysis; however, this effect may wear off after fluids are stopped if adequate hydration is not maintained. Caution must be exercised with multiple fluid boluses during labor, especially in the setting of patients with preeclampsia or patients on magnesium sulfate for any reason, due to the increased risk for pulmonary edema, as well as in the setting of patients on oxytocin due to the antidiuretic effect of oxytocin and the risk for water toxicity.

Oxygen Administration

Maternal oxygen administration, along with maternal position changes, has historically been among the most frequently performed intrauterine resuscitation techniques. The benefit of maternal oxygen administration has been debated for decades, and no clear consensus exists. Under normal conditions, the supply of oxygen is approximately twice fetal demand; therefore, fetal oxygen uptake is not affected until the maternal oxygen supply is cut in half (Reddy et al., 2021). Research suggests that while fetal hypoxia is not directly linked to maternal hypoxia, maternal oxygen supplementation results in increased free radicals in fetal circulation that may have adverse effects, including fetal cellular damage (Klinger et al., 2005). Multiple research studies have shown that while maternal oxygen administration may improve fetal hypoxia, it will not correct acidosis and does not provide fetal benefit (Fawole & Hofmeyr, 2012). A 2021 study evaluating use of supplemental oxygen found that there was no effect on umbilical artery pH or improvement of FHR tracing in low-risk patients; rather, it resulted in worsening of umbilical artery pH at delivery (Chuai et al., 2022). Based on the available literature, maternal oxygen supplementation should be reserved for maternal hypoxia. Administration for nonreassuring fetal status is not supported by current evidence (Hamel et al., 2014). A recent American College of Obstetricians and Gynecologists (ACOG) practice bulletin also recommends against the routine use of maternal oxygen supplementation in patients with normal oxygen saturation for fetal intrauterine resuscitation (ACOG, 2022).

Amnioinfusion

Amnioinfusion consists of the use of an intrauterine pressure catheter to replace fluid into the uterine cavity in an attempt to resolve variable decelerations by alleviating pressure on the umbilical cord (ACOG, 2009; ACOG & Society for Maternal-Fetal Medicine, 2023). Since ruptured membranes are required, this is not an option for a patient with intact amniotic membranes who is not in labor or undergoing induction of labor. As amnioinfusion is an invasive intervention, it is typically used as a second-line therapy for recurrent variable decelerations that do not improve with maternal position changes. It is not an indicated intervention specifically to dilute thick, meconium-stained fluid (ACOG, 2009). The literature supports the use of amnioinfusion for suspected umbilical cord compression related to the potential considerable neonatal benefit of improving umbilical artery pH at delivery (Hofmeyr & Lawrie, 2012). There is also evidence suggesting decreased Cesarean rates in the setting of recurrent variable decelerations (Kilpatrick & Papile, 2017). It is not indicated for the treatment of chorioamnionitis (Hofmeyr & Kiiza, 2016). Use should be limited to treatment of recurrent variable decelerations (ACOG, 2009, 2006). Potential complications include uterine overdistention, uterine hypertonus, infection, and amniotic fluid embolism. Contraindications include active maternal infection such as chorioamnionitis, HIV, or genital herpes; uterine anomalies; known or suspected placenta previa; malpresentation; overt nonreassuring fetal monitoring where a delay could compromise fetal status; and impending birth (Petrie, 2008).

General guidelines for amnioinfusion include informed consent before starting an amnioinfusion. Prior to initiation, a cervical exam should be performed to rule out prolapsed umbilical cord and assess fetal presentation and cervical dilation. The baseline uterine resting tone should also be noted. Room-temperature normal saline or lactated Ringer's solution is instilled into the uterus via intrauterine pressure catheter, beginning with a 250- to 500-mL bolus over 20 to 30 minutes via pump or gravity, followed by a continuous infusion of 2 to 3 mL/min for up to 1 L. Continuous fetal monitoring is required during amnioinfusion. If recurrent variable decelerations persist after 1 L amnioinfusion, it is considered a failed intervention and alternative therapies should be considered. If the uterine resting tone becomes persistently elevated, the amnioinfusion should be discontinued to allow the uterine pressure to equilibrate over approximately 5 minutes. An amnioinfusion should also be discontinued if the new resting tone is 15 mmHg above baseline or above 30 mmHg. Clinicians should note the amount of fluid instilled in comparison with the amount of fluid returned, and amnioinfusion should be stopped if uterine overdistention occurs so as to not increase the patient's overall risk for postpartum hemorrhage.

INTERVENTIONS RELATED TO ANESTHESIA-RELATED HYPOTENSION

Regional anesthesia increases the risk of supine hypotension, particularly immediately post placement. FHR abnormalities, including late decelerations or fetal bradycardia, may result. Initial interventions should include maternal position changes and IV fluid bolus. If unsuccessful, ephedrine or phenylephrine should be considered to increase vascular tone and maternal blood pressure. Ephedrine is the medication of choice and has not been associated with adverse fetal outcomes despite crossing the placenta (ACOG, 2019). In the event that terminal bradycardia results from maternal hypotension after regional anesthesia placement, an emergent cesarean delivery is indicated.

Clinical Pearl

Strong working relationships with anesthesia providers are key in the rapid identification and treatment of maternal hypotension secondary to regional anesthesia.

MODIFIED MATERNAL PUSHING EFFORTS IN THE SECOND STAGE OF LABOR

It is not uncommon to see category II fetal tracings during the second stage of labor. While most fetuses tolerate decelerations during the second stage, clinicians must consider that this is also a physiologically stressful period for the fetus under ideal circumstances. In comparison to passive fetal descent or "laboring down," active maternal pushing efforts lead to more FHR decelerations. By delaying maternal pushing efforts until the patient has the urge to push, the active pushing phase is shortened, and decelerations may be decreased (Simpson & James, 2005). While delayed pushing is standard practice in many facilities, evidence suggests that it has not been shown to increase the likelihood of vaginal delivery; risks including infection, hemorrhage, and neonatal acidemia should be discussed with the patient (ACOG, 2019). Sustained closed-glottis pushing and pushing for more than four times with each contraction should be avoided. Instead, consider three to four pushes per contraction lasting 6 to 8 seconds in order to facilitate both maternal and fetal well-being (Simpson, 2021).

In patients with deep, repetitive, and/or prolonged variable decelerations, the compromised, reduced uterine profusion related to either frequent contractions with minimal resting tone or prolonged maternal pushing efforts may lead to fetal acidosis. Prompt identification and intervention are essential. In patients with a prolonged deceleration, the decision to "outrun fetal distress" by urging continued pushing may only increase risks related to poor fetal oxygenation. Instead, consider allowing the fetus time to respond and recover before maternal pushing efforts resume. If the tracing was previously abnormal, recovery is considered unlikely, and immediate delivery via either continued maternal pushing efforts or operative delivery is indicated (Schifrin et al., 2022).

▶ INTERVENTIONS FOR FETAL HEART RATE ARRHYTHMIAS

Occasionally, FHR arrhythmias require intervention in utero. Treatment is often complex and multifactorial, with a multidisciplinary team approach. The most common fetal tachyarrhythmia requiring treatment is supraventricular tachycardia (SVT) with a range from 220 to 240 beats per minute (bpm). This rapid heartbeat increases the workload of the fetal heart, increases oxygen demand, and decreases cardiac output. If SVT persists more than 50% of the time, fetal oxygen demands may go unmet and lead to the development of congestive heart failure. Nonimmune fetal hydrops and fetal death may result. The severity of the fetal hydrops directly correlates with the severity of the hemodynamic compromise as well as fetal gestational age. The primary goal of therapy is the prevention or improvement of fetal hydrops through conversion to sinus rhythm or ventricular rate control. Successful conversion typically occurs 65% to 95% of the time within 1 week in the hydropic fetus or within 48 hours in the nonhydropic fetus (Wacker-Gussmann et al., 2014).

Treatment of fetal SVT varies greatly and can be highly successful. Observation is often the primary choice when the pregnancy is near term, episodes are short in duration, and there is no evidence of fetal hemodynamic compromise. Delivery is indicated in a fetal SVT at term without hydrops. Flecainide and digoxin are superior to sotalol in converting SVT to sinus rhythm (Jaeggi & Nii, 2005). Digoxin is recommended as first-line therapy in a nonhydropic fetus and may be loaded intravenously or orally (Zoller, 2017). IV loading is recommended to due quicker onset and more consistent absorption over oral loading doses; however, IV loading doses require closing maternal and fetal monitoring. Once fetal conversion has occurred, the pregnant patient can be switched to the oral form for maintenance. It is important to note that the digoxin dosage may need to be upward of twice the normal dose for a nonpregnant adult. Maternal digoxin levels should be monitored with a target therapeutic range of .8 to 2.0 ng/mL (Api & Carvalho, 2008). Flecainide is considered the most effective second-line therapy for successful conversion to sinus rhythm when digoxin has failed (Zoller, 2017). The hydropic fetus with SVT continues to present the most challenges. Digoxin alone may be ineffective and may require adding further medications such as flecainide, sotalol, or amiodarone. Sridharan et al. (2016) showed that in the hydropic fetus with SVT, flecnode is superior to digoxin; however, no universal consensus exists.

Fetal atrial flutter is the second most common fetal tachyarrhythmia, accounting for approximately 25% to 30% of cases. Of these cases, approximately 13% will go on to develop nonimmune fetal hydrops as a result (Jaeggi et al., 2011). Atrial flutter typically results from myocarditis, structural cardiac disease, and Sjögren's syndrome A (SSA) isoimmunization and occurs later in gestation. Currently, digoxin and sotalol are the treatments of choice, with sotalol being first-line in the hydropic fetus (Wacker-Gussmann et al., 2014). Flecainide and amiodarone have not been found to be safe or effective (Zoller, 2017).

Sinus bradycardia requires identification of any underlying causes and determination of fetal well-being. Management depends on the underlying pathology, gestational age, and overall fetal well-being. Mild fetal bradycardia (FHR of 100–110 bpm) may be seen in a postterm fetus secondary to a more mature parasympathetic branch of the autonomic nervous system. As long as the tracing remains >100 bpm with moderate variability with no declarations and no identifiable underlying pathology exists, continued observation with notification of the primary provider is acceptable. Sinus bradycardia with absent variability is a category III tracing and requires immediate corrective measures with a plan for expedited delivery (Macones et al., 2008).

Atrioventricular (AV) blocks occur in approximately 1 in 15,000 live births and are categorized as first, second, and third degree depending on their severity (Carvalho, 2019). Approximately 40% occur in cases with congenital cardiac malformations, particularly heterotaxy, or transposition of the great vessels. The remaining 60% are typically immune-mediated secondary to maternal connective tissue disorders (Abuhamad & Chaoui, 2016). First-degree blocks are difficult to diagnose and are not visible on an EFM tracing because the FHR is normal. Second-degree blocks are commonly caused by maternal collagen vascular disease and fetal congenital defects. Third-degree blocks are caused by cardiac structural defects, such as transposition of the great vessels, fetal cytomegalovirus, antiphospholipid antibody syndrome, and presence of maternal anti-SSA/Ro or anti-Sjögren's syndrome B (SSB)/La antibodies, such as are found in Sjogren's syndrome and occasionally lupus. Up to 50% of fetuses with a third-degree heart block will also have congenital cardiac disease (Jaeggi et al., 2011).

There is currently no consensus on the treatment of fetal heart block. Steroids that cross the placenta, particularly betamethasone and dexamethasone, have been suggested if the patient has a high anti-SSA/Ro or anti-SSB/La antibody titer in an effort to decrease inflammation and improve fetal cardiac function but should not be given if there is any specific contraindication to their use (Bravo-Valenzuela et al., 2018). When the ventricular rate falls below 50 bpm, hydrops becomes more common. Fetal hydrops creates additional management challenges with overall poor outcomes. Baseline FHR above 55 bpm, absence of cardiac structural defects, and absence of fetal hydrops improve the overall neonatal prognosis (Jaeggi et al., 2011). Following delivery, clinicians should be prepared for placement of a temporary pacemaker with consideration of permanent pacemaker placement.

Fetuses with cardiac arrhythmias often tolerate labor and may undergo a vaginal delivery as long as EFM is consistent with adequate oxygenation. In a fetus with premature atrial contractions only, treatment is often not indicated and does not require care in a tertiary facility. However, other fetal arrhythmias requiring intervention should undergo labor and delivery in a tertiary facility equipped to handle any complications that might arise during labor or immediately after delivery. If neonatal pacing or cardiac surgery is anticipated, delivery should be scheduled and appropriate interdisciplinary planning should occur in advance at a comprehensive facility.

▶ INTERVENTIONS FOR UTERINE PATTERN ABNORMALITIES

When managing labor patients, it is important to monitor uterine activity closely to avoid tachysystole when possible. Tachysystole has the potential to affect fetal oxygenation, particularly when it is oxytocin induced, because of maternal blood flow interruption during contractions (Leathersich et al., 2018). It is also one of the most common causes of fetal hypoxia and acidosis (Ayres-de-Campos et al., 2015). By allowing periods of adequate resting tone, there is more time for adequate placental perfusion and fetal oxygenation. Consideration must also be given to monitoring resting tone as a method for monitoring for complications such as placental abruption, by either clinician palpation or intrauterine pressure catheter.

As a contraction begins, the fetal reserve from the intervillous space is utilized while placental perfusion is impaired. A healthy, noncompromised fetus will tolerate this well with little to no recourse. Previous research suggests that fetal oxygenation saturation ($FSpO_2$) decreases during contractions, reaches its lowest level at approximately 92 seconds, and takes approximately 90 seconds to recover (McNamara & Johnson, 1995). When deciding on interventions related to uterine pattern abnormalities, it is imperative to consider the accompanying EFM tracing. The presence or absence of FHR abnormalities associated with uterine contractions is key to the identification of appropriate management. A secondary consideration is whether or not tachysystole is the result of spontaneous labor versus the result of oxytocin administration.

In patients with spontaneous labor, tachysystole, and category I FHR tracing, no intervention is required; however, the clinician should consider placing the patient in the lateral position to increase uteroplacental perfusion. In patients with spontaneous labor, tachysystole, and category II or III FHR tracing, intrauterine resuscitation measures should be implemented, with tocolysis consideration if intrauterine resuscitation measures fail (ACOG, 2009).

In patients with oxytocin-induced tachysystole and category I FHR tracing, the clinician should consider decreasing uterotonics. In patients with oxytocin-induced tachysystole and category II or III FHR tracing, uterotonics should be decreased or stopped, with intrauterine resuscitation measures initiated concurrently. Tocolytic agents should be considered if intrauterine resuscitation measures fail (ACOG, 2009).

UTERINE TOCOLYSIS

Uterine tocolytic agents are used on the premise of inhibition of uterine smooth muscle activity, with the assumption that this relaxation improves placental perfusion. Improved placental perfusion increases the likelihood of adequate fetal oxygenation. Tocolytics may be used to improve nonreassuring fetal heart tracings in an effort to facilitate vaginal delivery or to improve fetal status while preparing for operative delivery. Appropriate use may also decrease Cesarean section rates, as nonreassuring fetal tracings are one of the leading indications for an unplanned Cesarean section (Leathersich et al., 2018).

Reduction of uterine contraction frequency may be achieved in a variety of ways, including decreasing or discontinuing oxytocin, administering IV fluids, and/or administering tocolytics. Use of tocolytics should be considered a temporary measure for prolonged deceleration or nonreassuring fetal status. The recent literature suggests that there is insufficient evidence from multiple randomized controlled trials to determine the exact effects of tocolytics for tachysystole or nonreassuring fetal status during labor (Leathersich et al., 2018). Acute tocolysis may be considered in any situation where the continuation of even normal uterine activity may worsen fetal status or oxygenation. Approximately 20% of poor intrapartum outcomes are related to induction and/or augmentation issues (Sukumaran et al., 2020).

Several common medications are used for uterine tocolysis, including calcium channel blockers (specifically nifedipine), nonsteroidal antiinflammatory drugs (specifically indomethacin), beta-adrenergic agonists (specifically terbutaline), and magnesium sulfate. Each of these presents its own set of maternal and fetal adverse effects as well as unique contraindications. Nitroglycerine is also used in some facilities; however, compared with terbutaline, it has a significant impact on maternal blood pressure and is overall less effective. It is also important to remember that if a patient is receiving magnesium sulfate for fetal neuroprotection and continues to experience preterm labor, calcium channel blockers and beta-adrenergic agonists must be used with caution. Indomethacin may be used in conjunction with magnesium sulfate prior to 32 weeks' gestation for short-term treatment of preterm labor after potential risks and benefits are weighed (ACOG, 2009).

One of the most common tocolytics used is subcutaneous terbutaline, a beta$_2$-adrenergic agonist. A 2006 study suggests that oxytocin does not necessarily have to be stopped to give terbutaline. While this seems counterintuitive, oxytocin discontinuation involves a significant delay in the labor process. This study suggests that the administration of terbutaline concurrently with oxytocin continuation appears to be more effective for resolving tachysystole during labor without disrupting the normal labor process. There was no increase in fetal acidosis, significant differences in chorioamnionitis, or need for operative vaginal delivery using this technique. Average time to tachysystole resolution was 9 minutes 35 seconds with a lower rate of tachysystole recurrence in the group that received terbutaline while continuing oxytocin (Pacheco et al., 2006). Current recommendations for terbutaline dosing are .25 mg every 15 minutes for up to three doses, although variations to this regimen exist in clinical practice. Because terbutaline binds to beta$_1$ receptors at multiple sites, maternal tachycardia and hypotension may occur along with side effects such as palpitations, shortness of breath, headache, and nasal congestion. Patients may also develop hypokalemia and hyperglycemia. The maternal heart rate should be assessed and documented prior to administration. Terbutaline administration is contraindicated in patients with heart disease, hemorrhage, hypovolemia, and/or heart rate >120 beats per minute. It is also rarely associated with pulmonary edema, symptomatic arrhythmias, myocardial infarction, and death (Haas et al., 2014). Preemptive patient education related to potential side effects is vital prior to terbutaline administration.

While routinely used in obstetric practice, terbutaline for the prevention or treatment of preterm labor and uterine tachysystole remains off-label. The only U.S. Food and Drug Administration (FDA)–approved drug for tocolysis is ritodrine; however, is it no longer marketed in the United States. In 2011, the FDA published a warning that terbutaline should not be used for the prevention or prolonged treatment (beyond 48–72 hours) of preterm labor secondary to the potential for serious maternal cardiac complications and death (U.S. Food and Drug Administration, 2011). This warning was reaffirmed in 2017 and is supported by ACOG. Other studies report possible deleterious behavioral effects in children exposed to beta-adrenergic receptor agonists in utero (Witter et al., 2009). While short-term use may allow for antenatal corticosteroid administration and benefit as well as magnesium sulfate for neuroprotection, no evidence exists that tocolytic therapy has any favorable effect on neonatal outcomes (ACOG, 2009).

In the setting of threatened preterm labor, current ACOG recommendations advise against the prophylactic use of tocolytics in patients with preterm contractions without cervical change, especially those dilated <2 cm (2017, reaffirmed 2020). The upper limit for tocolytic use for the prevention of preterm delivery remains 34 weeks. It is imperative for clinicians to be keenly aware of contraindications to tocolysis, including intrauterine fetal demise, lethal fetal anomalies, nonreassuring fetal status, severe preeclampsia or eclampsia, maternal bleeding with hemodynamic instability, and chorioamnionitis (ACOG, 2009).

▶ KEY POINTS

- While the left lateral position is ideal for improving and promoting fetal circulation, other positions may be necessary to improve overall fetal status depending on the clinical situation.
- Maternal oxygen supplementation should be reserved for maternal hypoxia, as there is no fetal benefit and it may actually worsen fetal acidosis.
- The goal of intrauterine resuscitation and interventions related to fetal monitoring abnormalities is to prevent or reverse fetal hypoxia and acidosis.
- While not all fetal arrhythmias require intervention, understanding the role of the clinician for each allows for prompt assessment and intervention when required to prevent sequela, such as fetal hydrops.
- Careful and appropriate use of tocolytics is imperative to improve fetal outcomes and prevent fetal harm.

CASE STUDY

Emily is a 31-year-old G1P0 at 35 weeks and 1 day's gestation presenting to obstetric triage for extended fetal monitoring for suspected fetal tachycardia noted during the last two prenatal visits. Emily has no underlying medical history. Labs include complete blood count, comprehensive metabolic panel, thyroid-stimulating hormone, and free T_4. All labs are unremarkable. After 3 hours of the EFM tracing shown in the following, maternal-fetal medicine (MFM) is consulted for recommendations. An ultrasound is performed and confirms the absence of fetal hydrops.

Answer the following, and then see the "Case Study Answers" for correct answers.

1. Baseline FHR: _____

2. Variability: _____

3. Accelerations: Present or absent?

4. Decelerations
   a. Early: Present or absent?
   b. Variable: Present or absent?
   c. Late: Present or absent?
   d. Prolonged: Present or absent?

5. Contractions
   a. Frequency: _____
   b. Duration: _____

6. Interpretation: Category _____

7. Discuss all possible underlying causes for this tracing.

8. Determine priority actions and interventions based on the MFM diagnosis of persistent fetal tachycardia without fetal hydrops.

(*See answers next page.*)

CASE STUDY ANSWERS

1. Baseline FHR: 180 bpm

2. Variability: Moderate

3. Accelerations: Absent

4. Decelerations:
   a. Early: Absent
   b. Variable: Absent
   c. Late: Absent
   d. Prolonged: Absent

5. Contractions
   a. Frequency: None
   b. Duration: N/A

6. Interpretation: Category II

7. Possible underlying causes for this tracing include the following:
   - Maternal hyperthyroidism
   - Fetal anemia
   - Fetal distress
   - Maternal or fetal infection
   - Maternal fever
   - Maternal use of stimulants
   - Maternal dehydration
   - Fetal arrhythmia

8. Priority actions and interventions based on the MFM diagnosis of persistent fetal tachycardia without fetal hydrops include the following:
   - Administration of digoxin
   - Extended fetal monitoring
   - Admission to monitor maternal and fetal response to medication

KNOWLEDGE CHECK: CHAPTER 7

1. A preterm fetus with persistent tachycardia that is not hydropic is best treated with maternal administration of:
   A) Digoxin
   B) Phenobarbital
   C) Terbutaline

2. Amnioinfusion is recommended for a fetal heart rate (FHR) pattern with recurrent decelerations that are:
   A) Early
   B) Late
   C) Variable

3. The clinician notes a pattern of decelerations on the fetal monitor that begins shortly after the contraction and returns to baseline just before the contraction is over. The correct action by the clinician is to:
   A) Administer oxygen by face mask at 8 to 10 L/min
   B) Continue to monitor and record the normal pattern
   C) Position the patient on the left side

4. The clinician notes variable decelerations to 70 beats per minute (bpm) during the first stage of labor in a patient with intact amniotic membranes. The *initial* action should be:
   A) Fetal scalp stimulation
   B) Maternal oxygen administration
   C) Maternal position changes

5. The primary goal of treatment for late decelerations is to:
   A) Decrease cord compression
   B) Improve maternal oxygenation
   C) Maximize uteroplacental blood flow

6. An appropriate initial intervention for the following tracing shown during the first stage of labor is:

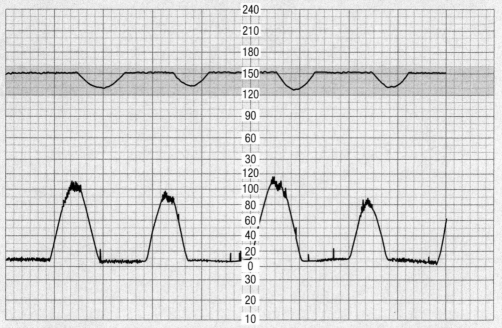

   A) Amnioinfusion
   B) Maternal repositioning
   C) Oxygen at 10 L via nonrebreather face mask

(*See answers next page.*)

1. A) Digoxin

Digoxin is the first-line treatment of persistent tachycardia without a hydropic fetus. Terbutaline is indicated for tocolysis. Phenobarbital has been historically used for eclamptic seizures.

2. C) Variable

The purpose of an amnioinfusion is to alleviate cord compression, which is the causative agent of variable decelerations. Early decelerations do not necessitate intervention. Late decelerations have uteroplacental causes and are not improved by amnioinfusion.

3. B) Continue to monitor and record the normal pattern

The pattern is an early deceleration and is reassuring. No intervention is indicated for early decelerations.

4. C) Maternal position changes

The initial intervention to alleviate cord compression secondary to variable decelerations in a patient with intact amniotic membranes is maternal repositioning. There is no evidence supporting the use of maternal oxygen administration. Fetal scalp stimulation is not used with intact amniotic membranes.

5. C) Maximize uteroplacental blood flow

Late decelerations are the result of uteroplacental insufficiency and are best corrected through improvement of uteroplacental blood flow. Variable decelerations are the result of cord compression. There is no evidence to support the use of maternal oxygen supplementation as treatment of fetal heart rate (FHR) abnormalities.

6. B) Maternal repositioning

Late decelerations are the result of uteroplacental insufficiency. Maternal repositioning should be the first intervention in an attempt to improve uteroplacental blood flow. Amnioinfusion is indicated for improving variable decelerations. There is no current evidence or literature to support the use of maternal oxygen administration.

7. A patient receives terbutaline for an external cephalic version. Which of the following is an expected response of the fetal heart rate (FHR)?
   A) Decrease in variability
   B) Increase in baseline
   C) No change

8. For a patient admitted in spontaneous labor with tachysystole and a category I tracing, which of the following should be the clinician's *initial* intervention?
   A) Administer IV fluid bolus
   B) Assist the patient to a lateral position
   C) Discontinue oxytocin (Pitocin)

9. Plans of the healthcare team with a patient with a sinusoidal fetal heart rate (FHR) pattern may include:
   A) Kleinhauer–Betke stain
   B) Nonstress test
   C) Tocolytic administration

10. Resuscitative measures improve fetal variability, but the fetal heart rate (FHR) is still not reactive. The clinician attempts fetal scalp stimulation, knowing that a well-oxygenated fetus will likely respond to scalp stimulation with:
    A) Acceleration
    B) Deceleration
    C) Fetal movement

(See answers next page.)

7. B) Increase in baseline

Terbutaline is known to cause an increase in baseline, which may also lead to fetal tachycardia. It does not affect variability.

8. B) Assist the patient to a lateral position

In the setting of a category I tracing, oxytocin (Pitocin) discontinuation is not required. An IV fluid bolus is not indicated because no tocolysis is indicated given the category I tracing. Assisting the patient to the lateral position will allow for improved uteroplacental blood flow to maintain the category I tracing.

9. A) Kleinhauer–Betke stain

Because one of the most common causes of sinusoidal FHR is fetal anemia, use of the Kleinhauer–Betke stain allows for assessment of fetal-maternal hemorrhage, indicating significant fetal blood loss. Tocolytics are not indicated with a sinusoidal pattern. A nonstress test will not provide any additional information as to the cause of a sinusoidal pattern and is not the best intervention.

10. A) Acceleration

A well-oxygenated, nonacidotic fetus will likely respond to fetal scalp stimulation with an acceleration as a noninvasive alternative to fetal scalp sampling, especially during the first stage of labor. It is not uncommon to not have a positive scalp stimulation test, making it poor at ruling in or out fetal hypoxia during the second stage of labor.

▶ REFERENCES

Abuhamad, A., & Chaoui, R. (2016). *A practical guide to fetal echocardiography: Normal and abnormal hearts* (3rd ed.). Wolters Kluwer.

American College of Obstetrics and Gynecology. (2022). *ACOG practice advisory: Oxygen supplementation in the setting of category II or III fetal heart tracings.* https:// www.acog.org/clinical/clinical-guidance/practice-advisory/articles/2022/01/ oxygen-supplementation-in-the-setting-of-category-ii-or-iii-fetal-heart-tracings

American College of Obstetrics and Gynecology. (2009). ACOG practice bulletin 106. Intrapartum fetal heart rate monitoring: Nomenclature, interpretation, and general management principles. *Obstetrics and Gynecology, 114*(1), 192–202. https://doi.org/10.1097/AOG.0b013e3181aef106

American College of Obstetrics and Gynecology. (2006). ACOG committee opinion 346. Amnioinfusion does not prevent meconium aspiration syndrome. *Obstetrics and Gynecology, 108*(4), 1053. https://doi.org/10.1097/00006250-200610000-00048

American College of Obstetrics and Gynecology. (2019). ACOG committee opinion 766. Approaches to limit intervention during labor and birth. *Obstetrics and Gynecology, 133*(2), e164–e173. https://doi.org/10.1097/AOG.0000000000003074

American College of Obstetrics and Gynecology, & Society for Maternal-Fetal Medicine. (2023). *Obstetric care consensus: Safe prevention of the primary cesarean delivery.* American College of Obstetrics and Gynecology. https://www.acog.org/clinical/clinical-guidance/ obstetric-care-consensus/articles/2014/03/safe-prevention-of-the-primary-cesarean-delivery

Api, O., & Carvalho, J. (2008). Fetal dysthymias. *Best Practice & Research Clinical Obstetrics and Gynaecology, 22,* 31–48. https://doi.org/10.1016/j.bpobgyn.2008.01.001

Ayres-de-Campos, D., Spong, C. Y., Chandraharan, E., & FIGO Intrapartum Fetal Monitoring Expert Consensus Panel. (2015). FIGO consensus guidelines on intrapartum fetal monitoring: Cardiotocography. *International Journal of Gynaecology and Obstetrics: The Official Organ of the International Federation of Gynaecology and Obstetrics, 131*(1), 13–24. https://doi.org//10.1016/j .ijgo.2015.06.020

Bravo-Valenzuela, N., Rocha, L., Machado Nardozza, L., & Araujo Juior, E. (2018). Fetal cardiac arrhythmias: Current evidence. *Annals in Pediatric Cardiology, 11*(2), 148–163. https://doi .org/10.4103/apc.APC_134_17

Bullens, L., van Runnard Heimel, P. J., Pieter, J., van der Hout-van der Jagt, M., & Oei, S. (2015). Interventions for intrauterine resuscitation in suspected fetal distress during term labor: A systematic review. *Obstetrical & Gynecological Survey, 70*(8), 524–539. https://doi.org/10.1097/ OGX.0000000000000215

Carvalho, J. (2019). Fetal dysrhythmias. *Best Practice & Research Clinical Obstetrics and Gynaecology, 58,* 28–41. https://doi.org/10.1016/j.bpobgyn.2019.01.002

Chuai, Y., Jiang, W., Zhang, L., Chuai, F., Sun, X., Peng, K., Gao, J., Dong, T., Chen, L., & Yao, Y. (2022). Effect of long-duration oxygen vs room air during labor on umbilical cord venous partial pressure of oxygen: A randomized controlled trial. *American Journal of Obstetrics and Gynecology, 227*(4), 629.e1–629.e16. https://doi.org/10.1016/j.ajog.2022.05.028

Clark, S. L., Nageotte, M. P., Garite, T. J., Freeman, R. K., Miller, D. A., Simpson, K. R., Belfort, M. A., Dildy, G. A., Parer, J. T., Berkowitz, R. L., & D'Alton, M. (2013). Intrapartum management of category II fetal heart rate tracings: Towards standardization of care. *American Journal of Obstetrics and Gynecology, 209*(2), 89–97. https://doi.org/10.1016/j.ajog.2013.04.030

Fawole, B., & Hofmeyr, G. (2012). Maternal oxygen administration for fetal distress. *Cochrane Database of Systematic Reviews, 12,* CD000136. https://doi.org/10.1002/14651858.CD000136.pub2

Hamel, M., Anderson, B., & Rouse, D. (2014). Oxygen for intrauterine resuscitation: Of unproved benefit and potentially harmful. *American Journal of Obstetrics and Gynecology, 211*(2), 124–127. https://doi.org/10.1016/j.ajog.2014.01.004

Haas, D. M., Benjamin, T., Sawyer, R., & Quinney, S. K. (2014). Short-term tocolytics for preterm delivery: Current perspectives. *International Journal of Women's Health, 6,* 343–349. https://doi .org/10.2147/IJWH.S44048

Hofmeyr, G. J., & Kiiza, J. A. (2016). Amnioinfusion for chorioamnionitis. *The Cochrane Database of Systematic Reviews, 2016*(8), CD011622. https://doi.org/10.1002/14651858.CD011622.pub2

Hofmeyr, G. J., & Lawrie, T. A. (2012). Amnioinfusion for potential or suspected umbilical cord compression in labour. *The Cochrane Database of Systematic Reviews, 1*(1), CD000013. https://doi .org/10.1002/14651858.CD000013.pub2

Jaeggi, E., & Nii, M. (2005). Fetal brady- and tachyarrhythmias: New and accepted diagnostic and treatment methods. *Seminars in Fetal Neonatal Medicine, 10*(6), 504–514. https://doi.org/10 .1016/j.siny.2005.08.003

Jaeggi, E. T., Carvalho, J. S., De Groot, E., Api, O., Clur, S. A. B., Rammeloo, L., McCrindle, B. W., Ryan, G., Manlhiot, C., & Blom, N. A. (2011). Comparison of transplacental treatment of fetal supraventricular tachyarrhythmias with digoxin, flecainide, and sotalol: Results of a nonrandomized multicenter study. *Circulation, 124*(16), 1747–1754. https://doi.org/10.1161/ CIRCULATIONAHA.111.026120

Kilpatrick, S., & Papile, L. (Eds.). (2017). *Guidelines for perinatal care* (8th ed.). American Academy of Pediatrics & American College of Obstetrics & Gynecology.

Klinger, G., Beyene, J., Shah, P., & Perlman, M. (2005). Do hyperoxaemia and hypercapnia add to the risk of brain damage after intrapartum asphyxia? *Archives of Disease in Childhood: Fetal and Neonatal Edition, 90*(1), F49–F52. https://doi.org/10.1136/adc.2003.048785

Leathersich, S. J., Vogel, J. P., Tran, T. S., & Hofmeyr, G. J. (2018). Acute tocolysis for uterine tachy-systole or suspected fetal distress. *The Cochrane Database of Systematic Reviews, 7*(7), CD009770. https://doi.org/10.1002/14651858.CD009770.pub2

Macones, G., Hankins, G., Spong, C., Hauth, J., & Moore, T. (2008). The 2008 National Institute of Child Health and Human Development workshop report on electronic fetal monitoring: Update on definitions, interpretation, and research guidelines. *Obstetrics & Gynecology, 112*(3), 661–666. https://doi.org/10.1097/AOG.0b013e3181841395

McNamara, H., & Johnson, N. (1995). The effect of uterine contractions on fetal oxygen saturation. *BJOG: An International Journal of Obstetrics & Gynaecology, 102*(8), 644–647. https://doi.org/10 .1111/j.1471-0528.1995.tb11403.x

Pacheco, L., Rosen, M., Gei, A., Saade, G., & Hankins, G. (2006). Management of uterine hyper-stimulation with concomitant use of oxytocin and terbutaline. *Obstetrical & Gynecological Survey, 61*(12), 771–772. https://doi.org/10.1097/01.ogx.0000248818.73806.ee

Petrie, K. (2008). Intrapartum complications. In S. Ratcliffe, E. Baxley, M. Cline, & E. Sakornbut (Eds.), *Family medicine obstetrics* (3rd ed., pp. 454–499). Mosby. https://doi.org/10.1016/ B978-032304306-9.50021-5

Raghurman, N. (2020). Response to category II tracing: Does anything help? *Seminars in Perinatology, 44*(2), 151217. https://doi.org/10.1016/j.semperi.2019.151217

Reddy, U. M., Weiner, S. J., Saade, G. R., Varner, M. W., Blackwell, S. C., Thorp, J. M. Jr., Tita, A. T. N., Miller, R. S., Peaceman, A. M., McKenna, D. S., Chien, E. K. S., Rouse, D. J., El-Sayed, Y. Y., Sorokin, Y., Caritis, S. N., & Eunice Kennedy Shriver National Institute of Child Health and Human Development (NICHD) Maternal-Fetal Medicine Units (MFMU) Network. (2021). Intrapartum resuscitation interventions for category II fetal heart rate tracings and improve-ment to category I. *Obstetrics and Gynecology, 138*(3), 409–416. https://doi.org/10.1097/AOG .0000000000004508

Schifrin, B. S., Koos, B. J., Cohen, W. R., & Soliman, M. (2022). Approaches to preventing intrapar-tum fetal injury. *Frontiers in Pediatrics, 10*, 915344. https://doi.org/10.3389/fped.2022.915344

Simpson, K. (2021). Physiologic interventions for fetal heart rate patterns. In A. Lydon, & K. Wisner (Eds.), *Fetal heart monitoring principles and practices* (6th ed., pp. 155–184). Association of Women's Health, Obstetric, and Neonatal Nurses.

Simpson, K., & James, D. (2005). Efficacy of intrauterine resuscitation techniques in improving fetal oxygen status during labor. *Obstetrics and Gynecology, 105*(6), 1362–1368. https://doi.org/10 .1097/01.aog.0000164474.03350.7c

Sridharan, S., Sullivan, I., Tomek, V., Wolfenden, J., Škovránek, J., Yates, R., Janoušek, J., Dominguez, T. E., & Marek, J. (2016). Flecainide versus digoxin for fetal supraventricular tachy-cardia: Comparison of two drug treatment protocols. *Heart Rhythm, 13*(9), 1913–1919. https:// doi.org/10.1016/j.hrthm.2016.03.023

Sukumaran, S., Jia, Y., & Chandraharan, E. (2020). Uterine tachysystole, hypertonus, and hyper-stimulation: An urgent need to get definitions right to avoid intrapartum hypoxic-ischaemic brain injury. *Global Journal of Reproductive Medicine, 8*(2), 1–8. https://doi.org/10.19080/ GJORM.2021.08.555735

U.S. Food and Drug Administration. (2011, February 17). *FDA drug safety communication: New warnings against the use of terbutaline to treat preterm labor.* Drug Safety and Availability. https://www.fda.gov/drugs/drug-safety-and-availability/fda-drug-safety-communication -new-warnings-against-use-terbutaline-treat-preterm-labor

Wacker-Gussmann, A., Strasburger, J. F., Cuneo, B. F., & Wakai, R. T. (2014). Diagnosis and treatment of fetal arrhythmia. *American Journal of Perinatology, 31*(7), 617–628. https://doi.org/10 .1055/s-0034-1372430

Witter, F., Zimmerman, A., Reichmann, J., & Connors, S. (2009). In utero beta 2 adrenergic agonist exposure and adverse neurophysiologic and behavioral outcomes. *American Journal of Obstetrics and Gynecology, 201*(6), 553–559. https://doi.org/10.1016/j.ajog.2009.07.010

Zoller, B. (2017). Treatment of fetal supraventricular tachycardia. *Current Treatment Options in Cardiology, 19*(7), 7. https://doi.org/10.1007/s11936-017-0506-x

Clinical Communication and Professional Issues

Antay L. Waters

▶ INTRODUCTION

Between 2018 and 2021, communication errors were identified as the main cause in 72% of all perinatal deaths, while 34% of cases reported to The Joint Commission under its sentinel event–reporting policy included inadequate fetal monitoring as a root cause (Lippke et al., 2021). Common safety issues related to the use of electronic fetal monitoring (EFM) include staff with inadequate knowledge or training to correctly interpret EFM strips; intra- and interobserver variability in EFM interpretation; poor communication among team members and inconsistent use of terminology related to EFM interpretation; and fear of conflict, intimidation, and/or failure to function as a team. These issues may result in delayed or no response to abnormal EFM findings and may ultimately adversely affect maternal, fetal, and/or neonatal outcomes.

▶ OBJECTIVES

- Analyze the importance of clear, concise, and consistent communication related to EFM interpretation and interventions.
- Review key communication strategies for improving patient care.
- Discuss the potential legal and ethical implications related to the use of EFM.

▶ KEY TERMS

- **Debriefing:** Directed, intentional conversation used to answer questions about a recent event in order to improve patient safety or address potential threats to patient safety, not intended to cast blame but rather as process improvement
- **Negligence:** Failure to provide proper care; includes the concepts of duty, breach of duty, causation, and damages
- **Quality improvement:** Framework for systematic improvement, often seeking to establish standardized, evidence-based processes designed to improve patient safety and reduce variation between individuals

▶ COMMUNICATION AND DOCUMENTATION OF FETAL HEART MONITORING INFORMATION

To enhance perinatal safety, the Agency for Healthcare Research and Quality (AHRQ) established the AHRQ Safety Program for Perinatal Care and Perinatal Safety Toolkit. Through this program, several recommendations emerged in a concerted effort to improve overall perinatal quality, safety, morbidity, and mortality. The most universal of these efforts is the use of the standard National Institute for Child Health and Human Development (NICHD) nomenclature and three-tiered system for interpreting, communicating, and documenting EFM findings. This provides a common language for use among providers and staff to decrease variation in terminology and provide accurate communication between caregivers. The 2008 NICHD Workshop developed standardized nomenclature to use for describing fetal heart rate (FHR) and uterine contraction patterns. According to this standard, a complete description of an EFM tracing requires a qualitative and quantitative assessment of uterine contractions; baseline FHR; baseline FHR variability; presence of FHR accelerations and periodic or episodic FHR decelerations; and changes over time. (This system is discussed in detail in Chapter 6.) It is imperative to objectively document all conversations and interventions related to patient care in real time, including specific details of what is reported to the provider.

Situational awareness during use of EFM refers to all staff caring for the patient knowing what the patient's plan is through briefings and team management, being aware of what is going on and what is likely to happen next, and knowing what resources are available if needed. In the context of EFM, situational awareness is particularly relevant for category II tracings, where continued surveillance is often required before a definitive course of action can be determined. It is imperative that staff know what resources are available to them should the patient's status suddenly change.

EFFECTIVE COMMUNICATION TOOLS

Several highly effective communication tools exist to promote this critical component of perinatal care, including Situation, Background, Assessment, and Recommendation (SBAR); callouts; huddles; and closed-loop communication techniques. These tools are important elements of teamwork training for safe EFM use. Having a unit-established process for eliciting a rapid response for specific category III EFM findings requiring immediate action increases the likelihood of improved perinatal outcomes. These tools are part of a larger AHRQ program known as TeamSTEPPS® (Agency for Healthcare Research and Quality [AHRQ], 2019).

- *SBAR*: Communication tool used to give a concise, clear report in an emergency or during staff handoff that includes the SBARs from the clinician
- *Callouts*: Communication tool used to effectively convey critical information to group members simultaneously during an emergency
- *Huddles*: Communication tool designed to share and/or reinforce plans already in place with all members of the healthcare team involved in the care of the patient; particularly useful prior to invasive procedures
- *Closed-loop communication*: Communication tool characterized by the process of acknowledging received information with a verbal message, confirming that the message understood by the recipient was the intended message
- *CUS tool*: Communication tool that serves as a verbal alarm, empowering all members of the healthcare team to "stop the line." The key words of the CUS tool are Concern, Uncomfortable, and Safety:
  - I am Concerned.
  - I am Uncomfortable.
  - This is a Safety issue.

DEBRIEFING

Debriefing is an important component to all patient safety–related events and is designed to be nonjudgmental and confidential. Effective debriefing should be completed as soon as possible after an event to discuss both what went well and what can be improved as a team. The literature shows that effective debriefing can improve teamwork in real time. While it may seem difficult to find time for a debriefing, it is vital to the quality improvement process and improving team performance. These events are excellent learning opportunities and do not have to be long, typically 3 to 5 minutes. Effective debriefing includes all parties involved, as well as:

- Use of confidential, nonjudgmental approach
- Accurate description, discussion, and documentation of key events
- Analysis of why the event occurred, what went well, and what could be done better— focusing on the process, not on individual performance
- Discussing lessons learned and how to improve the process for the next time this event occurs
- Creating a plan for formal change and process improvement

Clinical Pearl

Effective communication is vital and an essential component to any patient safety program. Use of proven effective communication strategies decreases the risk for communication errors in high-risk environments.

▶ LEGAL AND ETHICAL ISSUES IN FETAL HEART RATE MONITORING

Clinicians, particularly nurses, are consistently rated as among the most ethical professions year after year by the American public according to Gallup polls. Individual values, beliefs, and personal philosophies play major roles in moral and ethical decision-making in the healthcare environment.

EFM interpretation and management is a common issue in litigation involving adverse outcomes in term pregnancies. According to the most recent American College of Obstetricians and Gynecologists (ACOG) professional liability survey, published in 2015, 73.6% of OB/GYN physicians have experienced at least one professional liability claim during their career, with 22.1% (up from 20.9% in 2012) of obstetric claims involving EFM (Carpentieri et al., 2015).

STANDARD OF CARE

The standard of care is defined as the behavior of an ordinary, responsible, or prudent clinician, regardless of role. Standard of care is determined by a variety of sources, including, but not limited to, institutional policies, procedures, bylaws, rules, and regulations; professional organizations that provide guidelines in the obstetric setting; evidence-based publications; and collaborative agreements (as required). Substandard care occurs when a member of the healthcare team fails to provide care that meets the accepted standard. In addition to providing substandard care, failing to respond in a timely manner is also not the standard of care and may be described as negligent, especially if breach of duty is confirmed.

It is imperative to have a well-thought-out and well-organized chain of command in place and written in institutional policy, reflecting the organizational structure from staff nurse to chief medical and nursing officers. Following the chain of command allows all members of the healthcare team to be heard and nonjudgmental discussions and decisions to occur in the best interest of the patient.

ETHICAL PRINCIPLES

One must consider the various ethical principles commonplace in healthcare. Ethical considerations may come in conflict with one another as consideration is made for both the pregnant patient and the fetus(es). It is vital that all members of the healthcare team communicate effectively with one another as well as the patient. This must be documented clearly and concisely. Use of the chain of command and the ethics committee are resources available to all members of the healthcare team when an ethical conflict arises.

Autonomy

Autonomy is the freedom of choice and the accepting of responsibility for one's choice. Autonomy allows patients the ability to make independent decisions. Clinicians must ensure that patients have all of the necessary information needed to make informed decisions. This is often complicated by outside influences such as the internet, social media, or family and friends. Examples of autonomy include the right to refuse any treatment or medication and patient confidentiality.

The legal right to self-determination through the Patient Self-Determination Act supports autonomy. It is the core of all medical decision-making in the United States. Assuming they are deemed competent, pregnant patients have the right to make decisions for themselves and their fetuses about the medical care and treatments they receive as long as those decisions are legal at the state and federal levels.

Beneficence and Nonmaleficence

The concept of beneficence requires that actions taken should be done in an effort to promote good. Clinicians are to act in the best interest of the patient. The associated concept of nonmaleficence requires that if no good can be done, at least do no harm. Given our complex healthcare network, all providers must remember that the first duty is to the patient, regardless of their ability to pay. Another element to consider is risk-benefit ratio, one of the most complex problems faced in healthcare. For every intervention and action, every provider must consider both the potential benefits to the pregnant patient and the fetus and the potential risks.

Justice

Justice requires the distribution of benefits and burdens to be equitable. Given the significant morbidity and mortality among minority populations, the concept of justice provides ethical guidance for decisions. While one part of social justice is to ensure that all races and ethnicities receive equal care, another part of seeking justice is promoting the financial sustainability of the healthcare system for the greater good of society. All clinicians are called to "choose interventions and care settings that maximize benefits, minimize harm, and reduce costs" (Smith et al., 2012).

INFORMED CONSENT AND REFUSAL OF MEDICAL TREATMENT

Informed consent is an essential component of obstetric care and involves effective provider–patient communication. Patients have the right to understand their medical condition, receive comprehensive disclosure of all treatment options, have an opportunity to ask any questions, and receive assistance in making decisions. Providers have a legal and ethical obligation to provide comprehensive information about the medical condition; recommended medical treatments; risks, benefits, and alternatives for recommended treatments; and potential adverse outcomes related to declining recommended treatments. Successful communication between patient and provider fosters trust and shared decision-making in the patient–provider relationship.

The informed consent process occurs when communication between patient and provider results in the patient's agreement to and authorization of specific medical interventions. According to the American Medical Association (2022), informed consent may be obtained from the patient or their legal proxy if the patient is unable to make medical decisions. These three key criteria define a patient's ability to make informed decisions:

- Assessment of the patient's ability to understand their medical diagnosis and the implications of the treatment and treatment alternatives and to make an independent, voluntary decision
- Presentation of all relevant information in an accurate, sensitive manner, including but not limited to the patient's diagnosis, purpose of recommended interventions, how the recommended interventions are completed, and risks and potential benefits of all options, including foregoing all options
- Complete documentation of the informed consent conversation and the patient's (or their proxy's) decision in the medical record

In the event of an emergency in which the patient is unable to make a decision and a proxy is unavailable, providers may initiate treatment without prior informed consent and inform the patient/proxy at the earliest possible opportunity.

If a patient is found to have the capacity to make medical decisions, a patient's right to refuse medical care is founded on the basic ethical principle of autonomy. Providers must not impose their own beliefs on patients in order to influence their decisions. Special circumstances may arise that create concerns surrounding capacity, including several populations with unique rules and exceptions such as intoxicated patients, psychiatric patients, hospice/end-of-life patients, and minors. Minors create a unique situation in the obstetric world. In all states, minors may receive care without parental consent if the treatment is related to evaluation and treatment for sexually transmitted infections (STIs), pregnancy prevention with contraception, or pregnancy-related care (Pirotte & Benson, 2021).

CONFIDENTIALITY

Twenty-first-century clinicians face increasing challenges related to respecting confidentiality. In a world where information is quickly shared, an increasing amount of information has become sensitive. The Health Insurance Portability and Accountability Act (HIPAA) of 1996 mandated the confidentiality of all healthcare information. The Health Information Technology for Economic and Clinical Health (HITECH) Act, enacted as part of the American Recovery and Reinvestment Act of 2009, requires the adoption of meaningful use of healthcare technology, including the electronic transfer and sharing of sensitive, protected healthcare information. The social media–rich environment serves as a minefield for healthcare workers. This includes everything from "friending" patients on social media, to posting photos even if no patients are directly identified, to writing about a workday at the hospital even if the hospital is not named—all of these may be considered HIPAA violations and result in disciplinary action, termination of employment, civil fines, or criminal charges.

As with any rule, exceptions exist. Examples of HIPAA exceptions include suspicion of physical or sexual abuse and criminal acts. While abuse should be reported to the appropriate welfare authorities, criminal acts are reported to and handled by the appropriate law enforcement agency. All clinicians must also be aware of applicable state and federal public health laws, such as the reporting of infectious diseases, including STIs.

Clinical Pearl

Obstetrics is a high-litigation specialty for all members of the healthcare team. Following procedures and standards of care will decrease (but not remove) the likelihood of an adverse event.

▶ PATIENT SAFETY AND QUALITY IMPROVEMENT IN FETAL HEART RATE MONITORING

Patient safety is always of utmost importance; however, in the obstetric setting, it becomes increasingly complex when more than one life is at stake. The key safety elements for EFM are organized into the following six overarching principles of patient safety derived from the AHRQ Safety Program for Perinatal Care: standardizing when possible, creating independent checks, learning from mistakes, simulation, teamwork training, and patient and family engagement.

Increasing staff use of NICHD nomenclature may be supported through unit policies in regard to training and certification. EFM training courses and certification are offered through several professional organizations, commercial entities, and local colleges or universities. Few studies have examined the isolated and independent effect of formal EFM training or certification on perinatal health outcomes, although many perinatal safety interventions include EFM courses or certification as one component of a multicomponent approach to improving perinatal quality and safety.

In addition to formal training or certification, other strategies may support staff use of standardized terminology. EFM "strip rounds" or "strip conferences" are periodic, multidisciplinary reviews of actual EFM strips from past patients for the purposes of teaching and learning in a team environment. The emphasis of strip rounds is on practicing the use of standardized terminology for describing and communicating the findings from the strip. Regular peer review with feedback for all staff (physicians, midwives, and staff nurses) who use and interpret EFM is another strategy that can be used to support use of standard nomenclature. Professional competency assessment through methods such as the C-EFM certification exam provides an evidence-based, validated tool for both staff competency and medical staff credentialing and privileging processes specific to EFM. These tools are another strategy for improving standardization of EFM interpretation and communication.

Simulation provides proven strategies for the healthcare team to enhance both individual skills and teamwork. Effective simulations include all disciplines potentially involved and occur in a safe, nonthreatening environment conducive to learning. Ideally, drills will occur prior to an event on a scheduled basis rather than being reactionary. Simulation promotes effective interprofessional collaboration and education as well as improves overall safety for all patients in the healthcare institution. Regular multidisciplinary simulation allows the growth of relationships and improved teamwork and communication (Abas & Juma, 2016). This relationship improvement helps lead to a just culture within a healthcare system.

JUST CULTURE

While fairly new to healthcare, just culture has been active in the aviation industry since the 1970s, when the shift from determining who made the error to what underlying factors contributed to the error occurred (Gerstle, 2018). While recognizing that some degree of human error is inevitable, a just culture also requires all clinicians to recognize that they are not immune to making errors. A true just culture employs an environment ripe for learning and engagement, particularly in the face of patient safety threats and healthcare-related errors. Establishing a just culture requires awareness by all parties, policy implementation supporting a just culture, and building of policies and procedures that support a just culture. By having a true just culture, all healthcare providers are more likely to report errors secondary to embedded trust in the healthcare system. The shift to a just culture is a slow process that takes place over years, not months. Recognizing the concerns of all parties while ensuring the alignment of perceptions related to just culture and trust can improve outcomes, increase employee satisfaction, and potentially decrease preventable medical errors (Paradiso & Sweeney, 2019).

ALARM FATIGUE

Alarm fatigue occurs when clinicians have repeated high exposure to medical device alarms, ultimately leading to desensitization, missed high-risk alarms, and delayed response time. Alarm fatigue has become an increasing concern as healthcare becomes more reliant on technology, including that alarms have more automated features. Clinicians are also faced with higher patient volumes requiring monitoring. To compound the situation, with increasing automation, there are also an increasing number of false or nonactionable alarms (Woo & Bacon, 2020). While medical alarms are designed to alert clinicians to potential problems, the literature also suggests that they can be potentially hazardous to patient safety, with the greatest contributing factor being the excessive number of alarms, upward of 900 per day (Bach et al., 2018). Since 2016, hospitals have been expected to establish policies and procedures for managing and prioritizing alarms, including increasing staff education related to alarm management (Woo & Bacon, 2020).

▶ KEY POINTS

- ■ Effective communication is critical to the overall safety and well-being of both the pregnant patient and the fetus, particularly related to EFM. Using the 2008 NICHD nomenclature provides a framework for success.
- ■ Obstetric providers at all levels use family-centered philosophy and evidence-based practice to provide quality, cost-effective care across the continuum.
- ■ EFM plays a significant role in litigation. Potential legal implications affect the care of both the pregnant patient and the fetus.
- ■ All clinicians must be knowledgeable about laws related to the care of patients and their families in the states where they practice, as well as policies specific to the healthcare institutions where they practice.

● CASE STUDY

A nurse is working in a labor and delivery unit in a small town. Sarah, the patient, is about to give birth to her fifth child. Normally, the patient would give birth at home; however, her blood pressure is high. Sarah is experiencing pain rated at 9/10 but declines an epidural. She believes that pain is something that should be tolerated. About 15 family members are present to watch the birth, including the patient's other children. Suddenly, the fetal monitor indicates a category III tracing, and an emergency Cesarean section is recommended. Because of her personal beliefs, Sarah refuses with the full support of her family.

Consider the following, and then see the following for answers.

1. Discuss the ethical principles and their implications for this patient and the clinicians.

2. Can Sarah refuse the emergency Cesarean section given that she is competent to make this decision? Why or why not?

(See answers next page.)

CASE STUDY ANSWERS

1. The ethical principles and their implications for this patient and the clinicians are as follows:
   - Autonomy—Sarah has freedom of choice. This also means that Sarah accepts responsibility for the consequences of her choice—both positive and deleterious. As clinicians, informed consent is imperative. Accepting a patient's decision is often the most difficult part, but it is essential.
   - Beneficence—Clinicians should take actions in an effort to promote positive outcomes. While the clinicians cannot force Sarah to have the emergent Cesarean section, they can advocate for her fetus.

2. Assuming Sarah is competent to make clinical decisions, it is within her rights to refuse any medical treatment because of patient autonomy, assuming the informed consent process has been followed. Clinicians should carefully document all conversations with Sarah and ensure that the appropriate paperwork, including refusal of treatment, is signed and included in the electronic health record. In some instances, the hospital ethics committee and/or the local legal system may become involved based on the rights of the fetus, depending on state laws. It is imperative for clinicians to know the applicable laws in the state of practice.

KNOWLEDGE CHECK: CHAPTER 8

1. Alarm fatigue is a serious concern and can be minimized by:
   A) Desensitizing clinicians to alarms
   B) Establishing levels of priority
   C) Using only audible alarms

2. Validation of competence implies:
   A) Demonstration of clinical skills while being observed by a preceptor
   B) Evaluation of level of knowledge and verification of clinical skills
   C) Validation of expertise by performance on formal examinations

3. A characteristic of a high-reliability perinatal unit is:
   A) Addressing of alarms only by leadership
   B) Creation of a just culture
   C) Reliance on protocol memorization

4. Who is responsible for the process of obtaining informed consent?
   A) Nurse
   B) Patient
   C) Physician/advanced practice provider

5. A nurse is caring for a patient who has a birth plan requesting that the neonate not receive any medications, including erythromycin ophthalmic ointment. Which ethical principle applies?
   A) Autonomy
   B) Beneficence
   C) Justice

6. When a clinician fails to uphold the expected legal and professional responsibilities, this is generally known as:
   A) Liability
   B) Malpractice
   C) Negligence

7. A healthcare worker has moved into a new community and will begin practicing. Why is it important for this healthcare worker to become familiar with the local community?
   A) It is not necessary to become familiar with the local community
   B) The health of the community impacts the health of its members
   C) The local community may use alternative treatment methods

8. A nurse overhears a colleague tell a patient that based on genetic testing results, the patient should terminate their pregnancy. What ethical principle has the clinician usurped?
   A) Autonomy
   B) Beneficence
   C) Justice

9. A nurse has an order to administer an IV bolus of penicillin but inadvertently gives an IV bolus of potassium. The nurse recognizes the error and realizes this is an example of:
   A) At-risk behavior
   B) Human error
   C) Reckless behavior

10. *Just culture* requires creating an environment that is:
    A) Judgmental
    B) Laissez-faire
    C) Open and fair

(See answers next page.)

1. B) Establishing levels of priority
Alarm fatigue is a real and present danger in the healthcare setting that requires attention. By establishing levels of priority, clinicians are able to determine which alarms require immediate attention. Using both audible and visual alarms reduces the risk of alarm fatigue. Desensitizing clinicians to medical alarms increases the risk for error because high-risk alarms may be overlooked or ignored.

2. B) Evaluation of level of knowledge and verification of clinical skills
Competency validation evaluates level of knowledge and verifies clinical skills through demonstration. Competency should not be based solely on formal exams or demonstration to a preceptor.

3. B) Creation of a just culture
Creation of a just culture increases the reliability and safety of the perinatal unit by facilitating an open and fair culture dedicated to learning and safe systems. Alarms being addressed only by leadership leaves room for error, alarm fatigue, and patient mismanagement. Memorizing protocols creates a patient safety hazard in the event that something occurs that does not exactly follow a protocol. It removes the ability of the clinician to think critically and provide the best care possible.

4. C) Physician/advanced practice provider
The physician or advanced practice provider performing the intervention is responsible for obtaining informed consent. Nurses are responsible for verification and witnessing of the appropriate signature as well as ensuring that the patient is of legal age and is competent to provide consent. The role of the patient is to make a fully informed decision based on the information provided.

5. A) Autonomy
Autonomy respects the patient's right to choose and requires the clinician to put their own opinions aside, even if they do not agree with the patient's decision. Beneficence requires that the clinician make decisions in the best interest of the patient. Justice requires the fair treatment of all individuals with the equitable allocation of resources.

6. B) Malpractice
Malpractice is any act or omission that deviates from the accepted norms and standards of care in the medical community. Negligence is failure to provide reasonable care, which may result in damages. Liability is the state of being responsible for something.

7. B) The health of the community impacts the health of its members
The epidemiology of a given area impacts the health of its community members. Awareness and ability to perform appropriate epidemiologic interventions will improve the health and well-being of the members of the community. While the local community may use alternative treatment methods, it is most important to understand the overall health of the community. Avoiding familiarity with the local community is a disservice to the patients served. Local, state, and national initiatives, such as *Healthy People 2030*, depend on community familiarity by healthcare workers to improve care and provide and add needed resources.

8. A) Autonomy
Autonomy respects the patient's right to choose and requires the clinician to put their own opinions aside. Beneficence requires that the clinician make decisions in the best interest of the patient. Justice requires the fair treatment of all individuals with the equitable allocation of resources.

9. B) Human error
Human error is an inadvertent action. At-risk behavior is a behavior choice made when the risk of the choice is not recognized. Reckless behavior is a behavioral choice with conscious disregard of substantial and unjustifiable risk.

10. C) Open and fair
Just culture requires creating an open and fair environment that is nonjudgmental, focusing on processes rather than individual faults. Just culture requires interventions at appropriate times with focus on process improvement rather than a laissez-faire approach.

▶ REFERENCES

Abas, T., & Juma, F. Z. (2016). Benefits of simulation training in medical education. *Advances in Medical Education and Practice, 7*, 399–400. https://doi.org/10.2147/AMEP.S110386

Agency for Healthcare Research and Quality. (2019). *TeamSTEPPS fundamentals course: Module 3. Communication.* https://www.ahrq.gov/teamstepps/instructor/fundamentals/module3/igcommunication.html

American Medical Association. (2022). *Informed consent.* American Medical Association Ethics. https://www.ama-assn.org/delivering-care/ethics/informed-consent

Bach, T., Berglund, L., & Turk, E. (2018). Managing alarm systems for quality and safety in the hospital setting. *BMJ Open Quality, 7*(3), e000202. https://doi.org/10.1136/bmjoq-2017-000202

Carpentieri, A., Lumalcuri, J., Shaw, J., & Joseph, G. (2015). *Overview of the 2015 American College of Obstetricians and Gynecologists' survey on professional liability.* American College of Obstetricians and Gynecologists. https://protectpatientsnow.org/wp-content/uploads/2016/02/2015PLSurveyNationalSummary11315.pdf

Gerstle, C. (2018). Parallels in safety between aviation and healthcare. *Journal of Pediatric Surgery, 53*(5), 875–878.

Lippke, S., Derksen, C., Keller, F., Kötting, L., Schmiedhofer, M., & Welp, A. (2021). Effectiveness of communication interventions in obstetrics—A systematic review. *International Journal of Environmental Research and Public Health, 18*(5), 2616. https://doi.org/10.3390/ijerph18052616

Paradiso, L., & Sweeney, N. (2019). Just culture. *Nursing Management, 50*(6), 38–45. https://doi.org/10.1097/01.NUMA.0000558482.07815.ae

Pirotte, B., & Benson, S. (2021). *Refusal of care.* StatPearls Publishing. https://www.ncbi.nlm.nih.gov/books/NBK560886/

Smith, C., & Alliance for Academic Internal Medicine-American College of Physicians High Value, Cost-Conscious Care Curriculum Development Committee. (2012). Teaching high-value, cost-conscious care to residents: The alliance for academic internal medicine-American College of Physicians curriculum. *Annals of Internal Medicine, 157*(4), 285.

Woo, M., & Bacon, O. (2020). Alarm fatigue. In K. K. Hall, S. Shoemaker-Hunt, L. Hoffman, S. Richard, E. Gall, E. Schoyer, D. Costar, B. Gale, G. Schiff, K. Miller, T. Earl, N. Katapodis, C. Sheedy, B. Wyant, O. Bacon, A. Hassol, S. Schneiderman, M. Woo, L. LeRoy, … A. Lim (Eds.), *Making healthcare safer III: A critical analysis of existing and emerging patient safety practices.* Agency for Healthcare Research and Quality.

Practice Test

Antay L. Waters

▶ PRACTICE TEST QUESTIONS

1. Fetal well-being is assessed during labor by evaluation of:
   A) Fetal heart rate (FHR) only
   B) FHR in relation to contractions
   C) Uterine contraction pattern

2. A clinician is explaining the purpose of electronic fetal monitoring (EFM). Which of the following statements accurately describes the purpose of EFM?
   A) EFM is a diagnostic procedure that monitors fetal heart rate (FHR) and contractions
   B) EFM is a screening procedure that monitors FHR and contractions
   C) EFM is a screening procedure that monitors only FHR

3. Fetal chemoreceptors are located in the:
   A) Aortic arch
   B) Carotid bodies
   C) Inferior vena cava

4. A patient presents for a term induction of labor with oligohydramnios. Based on this, a fetal heart rate (FHR) change that can be expected is:
   A) Early decelerations
   B) Late decelerations
   C) Variable decelerations

5. The patient is in early labor with oxytocin (Pitocin) infusing at 8 milliunits/minute and a category I tracing. Over the next 25 minutes, there are 28 uterine contractions, a change in fetal heart rate (FHR) tracing to category III, and new-onset heavy vaginal bleeding. Initial recommended management is to:
   A) Administer terbutaline
   B) Insert internal fetal monitors
   C) Prepare for Cesarean section

6. Late decelerations secondary to hypoxia are mediated primarily by:
   A) Baroreceptors
   B) Chemoreceptors
   C) Vagal response

7. While monitoring, the clinician recognizes that the baseline fetal heart rate (FHR) is identified as the average rate of a:
   A) 10-minute segment, excluding periodic or episodic changes
   B) 20-minute segment, excluding periodic or episodic changes
   C) 30-minute segment, excluding periodic or episodic changes

8. A term neonate is delivered, and arterial umbilical cord gases are obtained afterward. The results are as follows: pH of 7.05; partial pressure of carbon dioxide (pCO_2) of 75; partial pressure of oxygen (pO_2) of 23; bicarbonate (HCO_3) of 29; base excess of −11. What do these results indicate?
   A) Metabolic acidosis
   B) Mixed acidosis
   C) Respiratory acidosis

9. A patient desires a natural childbirth; however, the clinicians pressure the patient to have an epidural placed. This is an example of violation of which ethical principle?
    A) Autonomy
    B) Beneficence
    C) Justice

10. If an acceleration of the fetal heart rate (FHR) is elicited during scalp stimulation, the fetal pH can be assumed to be at least:
    A) 6.92
    B) 6.95
    C) 7.02

11. In a patient with oxytocin-induced tachysystole with a category I tracing, the *first* intervention should be to:
    A) Administer IV fluid bolus
    B) Discontinue the oxytocin (Pitocin)
    C) Help move the patient to a lateral position

12. In the United States, electronic fetal monitoring (EFM) paper speed is set at:
    A) 1 cm/min
    B) 2 cm/min
    C) 3 cm/min

13. If a patient were complete and pushing, which initial resuscitation measure would be appropriate?
    A) Amnioinfusion
    B) IV fluid bolus
    C) Modified pushing

14. When using the SBAR communication tool, the "R" involves:
    A) Making a recommendation
    B) Reporting lab results
    C) Reviewing medical history

15. In early pregnancy, the fetus compensates for decreased maternal circulating volume. The fetus does this by raising cardiac output via increasing:
    A) Fetal movement
    B) Heart rate
    C) Stroke volume

16. During a time of fetal stress with catecholamine release, blood flow is:
    A) Shunted away from the adrenal glands
    B) Shunted toward the adrenal glands
    C) Unchanged

17. The most common fetal tachyarrhythmia has absent-to-minimal variability and occurs at a rate of how many beats per minute (bpm)?
    A) 160 to 200
    B) 200 to 220
    C) 220 to 240

18. The fetal heart rate (FHR) pattern that can *most likely* be expected in postterm pregnancy includes:
    A) Early decelerations with moderate variability
    B) Marked variability
    C) Variable decelerations with occasional late decelerations

19. What is the *most common* cause of the following fetal monitoring tracing?

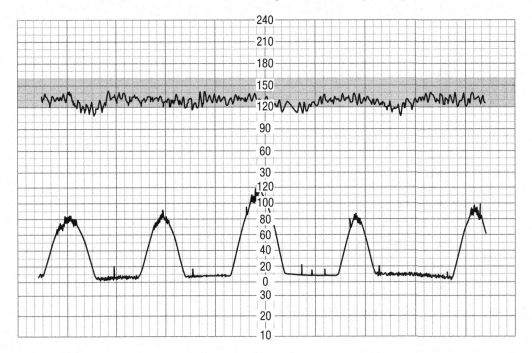

   A) Fetal head compression
   B) Umbilical cord compression
   C) Uteroplacental insufficiency

20. At 26 weeks, the fetal heart rate (FHR) baseline begins to decline. This is a normal physiologic response to the development of the:
   A) Baroreceptors
   B) Chemoreceptors
   C) Vagus nerve

21. The normal baseline fetal heart rate (FHR) is how many beats per minute?
   A) 100 to 160
   B) 110 to 160
   C) 120 to 160

22. The fetus has an intrinsic response to oxygen deprivation. Catecholamine levels increase, reducing peripheral blood flow while increasing blood flow to vital organs. How do these changes affect fetal blood pressure (BP) and fetal heart rate (FHR)?
   A) They decrease both BP and FHR
   B) They increase both BP and FHR
   C) They increase BP and decrease FHR

23. Significant neonatal morbidity occurs when more than how many minutes elapses between the onset of significant fetal heart rate (FHR) decelerations and delivery?
   A) 12
   B) 15
   C) 18

24. According to the National Institute of Child Health and Human Development (NICHD), fetal heart rate (FHR) decelerations that occur with <50% of contractions are:
   A) Intermittent
   B) Recurrent
   C) Repetitive

25. A pregnant patient in labor is currently being monitored externally but has a suspected fetal arrhythmia. The *next best* action is to:
    A) Employ a Doppler to listen to the ventricular rhythm
    B) Insert a fetal spiral electrode and turn off the logic
    C) Turn off the logic if an external monitor is in place

26. Which of the following is *not* considered a category III fetal tracing?
    A) Prolonged deceleration with absent variability
    B) Recurrent late decelerations with absent variability
    C) Recurrent late decelerations with minimal variability

27. Which of the following actions would be *best* to stimulate an acceleration in a patient with ruptured membranes?
    A) Making maternal position changes
    B) Performing a cervical exam
    C) Providing juice to the patient

28. A deceleration from 145 beats per minute (bpm) to 110 bpm for 14 minutes may be defined as a:
    A) Baseline change
    B) Late deceleration
    C) Prolonged deceleration

29. The clinician monitoring the fetal heart rate (FHR) pattern discovers that there is no variability accompanied by a smooth, undulating wave pattern. The nurse determines that the fetus can be placed in which of the following categories?
    A) Category I
    B) Category II
    C) Category III

30. Decreased intervillous exchange of oxygenated blood resulting in fetal hypoxia is typically present in which type of decelerations?
    A) Early
    B) Late
    C) Variable

31. Place the following interventions for a sinusoidal fetal heart rate (FHR) in the correct order:
    1. Prepare for Cesarean delivery.
    2. Place patient in lateral position.
    3. Determine if pattern is related to narcotic analgesic administration.
    A) 1, 2, 3
    B) 2, 3, 1
    C) 3, 2, 1

32. While the clinician is caring for a 145-kg laboring patient who is HIV positive, the external fetal heart rate (FHR) tracing is difficult to obtain. An appropriate nursing action would be to:
    A) Apply a fetal scalp electrode
    B) Auscultate for the presence of FHR variability
    C) Notify the attending physician or midwife

33. Bradycardia in the second stage of labor following a previously normal tracing may be caused by fetal:
    A) Hypoxemia
    B) Rotation
    C) Vagal stimulation

34. What is the most common cause of the following fetal monitoring tracing?

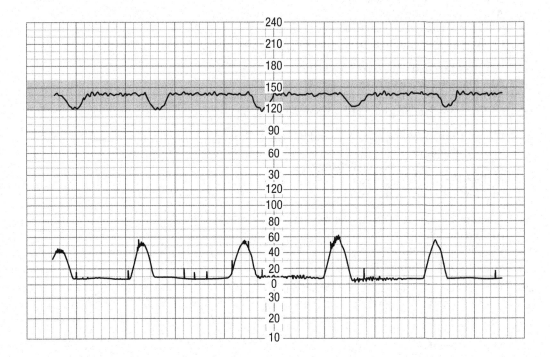

A) Fetal head compression
B) Umbilical cord compression
C) Uteroplacental insufficiency

35. The criteria for a fetal heart rate (FHR) acceleration after 32 weeks' gestation includes a rise in the FHR of *at least*:
A) 10 beats per minute (bpm) for at least 15 seconds
B) 15 bpm for at least 10 seconds
C) 15 bpm for at least 15 seconds

36. Findings indicative of progressive fetal hypoxemia are:
A) Late decelerations, moderate variability, and stable baseline rate
B) Loss of variability with recurrent late or variable decelerations
C) Prolonged decelerations recovering to baseline and moderate variability

37. A workup for maternal systemic lupus erythematosus would likely be ordered in the presence of:
A) Fetal heart block
B) Fetal supraventricular tachycardia
C) Premature ventricular contractions

38. Which IV fluid is most appropriate for intrauterine resuscitation?
A) .45% sodium chloride
B) .9% sodium chloride
C) 5% dextrose in .9% sodium chloride

39. Which of the following is *not* a probable cause of the following tracing shown?

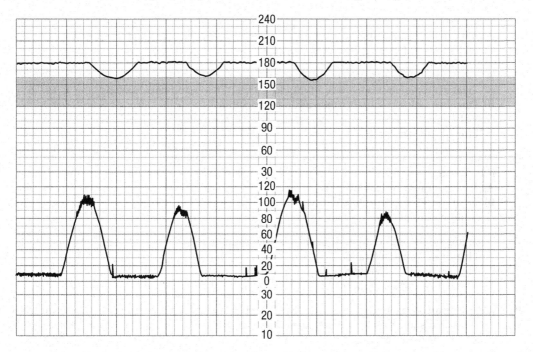

A) Fetal heart block
B) Maternal fever
C) Sympathomimetic drugs

40. The fetal heart rate (FHR) characteristic most predictive of a well-oxygenated fetus at the time observed is:
A) Absence of decelerations
B) Moderate variability
C) Stable baseline rate

41. During a hypoxic episode, fetal blood flow is shifted to the:
A) Brain
B) Liver
C) Lungs

42. A nurse wants to document a conversation with the attending physician that occurs during an emergent Cesarean section. The *best* approach to documenting the event would be to:
A) Continue providing care to the patient and write a late entry after the Cesarean section is complete
B) Enter an objective entry while colleagues prepare the patient for the Cesarean section
C) Report the conversation to the charge nurse, who can make an entry in the electronic health record

43. A 19-year-old G2P1001 patient is at 6 cm dilation and making good progress in labor with prolonged rupture of membranes. The patient has developed a fever of 102°F (38.89°C) and is now on antibiotics and acetaminophen (Tylenol). Which of the following statements is *accurate* in this case?
A) Cesarean delivery will prevent the fetus from developing sepsis
B) If there is fetal tachycardia that persists, the fetus is in imminent danger of developing heart failure
C) Maternal fever in the presence of fetal tachycardia does not necessarily require Cesarean delivery

44. An appropriate *initial* treatment for recurrent late decelerations with moderate variability during first-stage labor is:
    A) Amnioinfusion
    B) Maternal repositioning
    C) Oxygen at 10 L per nonrebreather face mask

45. Which of the following statements is *true*?
    A) Fetal hemoglobin has a lower affinity for oxygen than adult hemoglobin
    B) Fetal hemoglobin is higher than adult hemoglobin
    C) With an abrupt decrease in oxygen, the fetus compensates by redistributing blood to the brain, heart, and lungs

46. While most fetal dysrhythmias are not life-threatening, fetal supraventricular tachycardia (SVT) may lead to:
    A) Fetal complete heart block
    B) Fetal congestive heart failure
    C) Maternal congestive heart failure

47. What are the two most important characteristics to note when monitoring the fetal heart?
    A) Heart rate and accelerations
    B) Heart rate and variability
    C) Variability and accelerations

48. Following an ultrasound that revealed decreased amniotic fluid, a patient at term is admitted in early labor. It should be recognized that oligohydramnios often results in fetal heart rate (FHR) decelerations that are:
    A) Late in onset or occurring after the peak of the contraction
    B) Synchronous with the contraction
    C) Varied in depth and duration

49. Which of the following fetal systems has the greatest influence on fetal pH?
    A) Heart
    B) Kidneys
    C) Nervous system

50. Fetal scalp stimulation should be attempted when the fetal heart rate (FHR) is not reactive because a well-oxygenated fetus will respond with a(n):
    A) Baseline change
    B) Deceleration
    C) Acceleration

51. While using a fetal scalp electrode, the clinician notices an abnormally low fetal heart rate (FHR) on the monitor. What is the most appropriate *first* action?
    A) Calling the provider immediately
    B) Comparing maternal pulse with FHR
    C) Removing the fetal scalp electrode

52. Which of the following describes normal uterine activity?
    A) Frequency of 1 to 2 minutes
    B) Intensity of 100 mmHg in early labor
    C) Resting tone of less than 20 to 25 mmHg

53. A patient is admitted for induction of labor for preeclampsia with severe features. The fetal heart rate's (FHR's) variability might reflect routine management by:
    A) Decreasing
    B) Increasing
    C) Staying the same

54. The fetal heart rate (FHR) pattern characteristic of cephalopelvic disproportion, especially when seen during early labor, is decelerations that are:
    A) Early
    B) Late
    C) Variable

55. Baseline fetal heart rate (FHR) is determined over which period of time in minutes, excluding accelerations and decelerations?
    A) 10
    B) 20
    C) 30

56. Which of the following maternal medications could cause the following fetal heart rhythm shown?

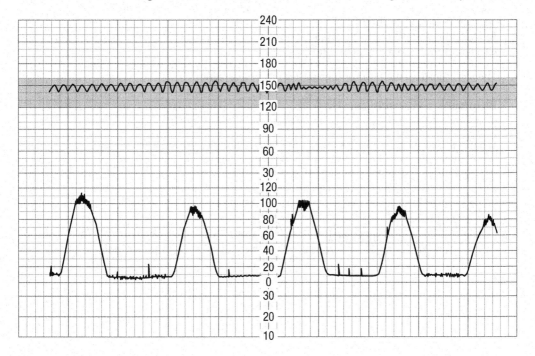

    A) Butorphanol
    B) Morphine
    C) Fentanyl

57. The recommended fetal heart rate (FHR) assessment interval for a low-risk patient with intermittent auscultation during the second stage of labor is every:
    A) 5 minutes
    B) 15 minutes
    C) 30 minutes

58. A patient at 38 weeks' gestation has had an uneventful labor with normal electronic fetal monitoring (EFM) tracings. Spontaneous rupture of membranes occurs, and the patient has a prolonged deceleration to 90 beats per minute. What is the first action?
    A) Amnioinfusion
    B) Cervical examination
    C) Maternal position changes

59. In the context of moderate variability, what type of decelerations are considered neurogenic in origin and amenable to intrauterine resuscitation techniques aimed at maximizing uterine blood flow?
    A) Early
    B) Late
    C) Variable

60. Monoamniotic-monochorionic twins are prone to what type of decelerations during labor?
    A) Early
    B) Late
    C) Variable

61. In a patient with oxytocin-induced tachysystole with an indeterminate electronic fetal monitoring (EFM) tracing, which of the following should be the *initial* intervention?
    A) Administering IV fluids
    B) Assisting the patient to right lateral position
    C) Discontinuing the oxytocin (Pitocin)

62. The *most* sensitive method for uterine activity assessment is:
    A) External tocotransducer
    B) Intrauterine pressure catheter
    C) Manual palpation

63. What is the *most* common cause of the following fetal monitoring tracing seen?

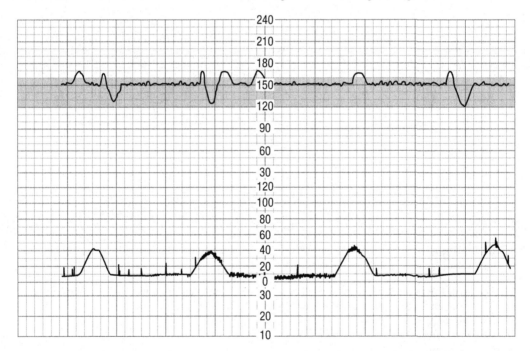

    A) Fetal head compression
    B) Umbilical cord compression
    C) Uteroplacental insufficiency

64. Which of the following is *not* a common cause for late decelerations?
    A) Collagen vascular disease
    B) Maternal diabetes mellitus
    C) Multifetal gestation

65. A tracing shows intermittent abrupt decelerations in a laboring patient. The *first* nursing action should be:
   A) Amnioinfusion
   B) Application of oxygen
   C) Maternal position changes

66. Resting tone and uterine contraction intensity *cannot* be accurately assessed by:
   A) External tocodynamometer
   B) Intrauterine pressure catheter
   C) Manual palpation

67. What should the *next* intervention be based on interpretation of the following strip?

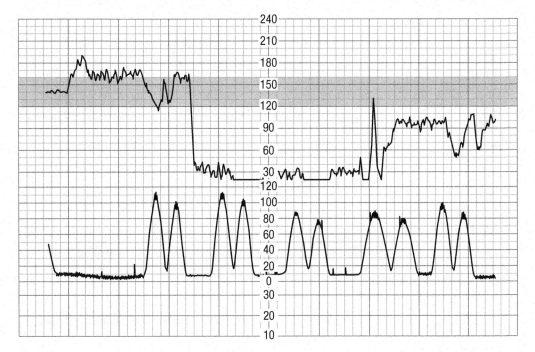

   A) Administer IV fluid bolus
   B) Administer magnesium sulfate (MgSO$_4$)
   C) Administer terbutaline (Brethine)

68. Which assessment or intervention would be *least* appropriate in a patient whose fetal heart rate (FHR) tracing reveals tachycardia and a prolonged deceleration?
   A) Assisting the patient to right lateral position
   B) Performing a cervical examination
   C) Performing fetal scalp stimulation

69. When the parasympathetic nervous system is stimulated, the fetal heart rate (FHR):
   A) Decreases
   B) Increases
   C) Stays the same

70. A patient is admitted with threatened preterm labor at 27 weeks' gestation and receives steroids in the event of preterm delivery. Which of the following changes may be transiently seen in this setting?
   A) Decrease in baseline
   B) Decrease in variability
   C) Increase in variability

71. Which of the following characteristics are most common in the preterm fetus?
    A) Increased baseline and prolonged accelerations
    B) Increased baseline and variable decelerations
    C) Prolonged accelerations and variable decelerations

72. What typical uterine activity characteristics may be present in preterm labor?
    A) Low-amplitude, high-frequency contractions
    B) Tetanic contractions
    C) Uterine irritability

73. Since widespread use of electronic fetal monitoring (EFM) began, the rate of cerebral palsy has:
    A) Gone down
    B) Gone up
    C) Not changed

74. In comparison with maternal blood, the affinity of fetal blood for oxygen is:
    A) Comparable
    B) Higher
    C) Lower

75. The *most frequently* encountered fetal heart rate (FHR) abnormality is decelerations that are:
    A) Early
    B) Late
    C) Variable

76. The *least likely* cause of fetal tachycardia is maternal:
    A) Fever
    B) Hyperthyroidism
    C) Hypothyroidism

77. Which of the following conditions is *not* an indication for antepartum fetal testing?
    A) Breech presentation
    B) Gestational diabetes
    C) Gestational hypertension

78. Amino acids, water-soluble vitamins, calcium, phosphorus, iron, and iodine are transferred across the placenta via:
    A) Active transport
    B) Passive diffusion
    C) Simple diffusion

79. Placement of the ultrasound transducer over which fetal part yields the *best* electronic fetal monitoring (EFM) recording?
    A) Back
    B) Chest
    C) Stomach

80. Which type of deceleration is *most likely* seen during the transitional phase of labor?
    A) Early
    B) Late
    C) Variable

81. All of the following are appropriate interventions for fetal tachycardia *except*:
    A) Assess maternal vital signs
    B) Increase maternal IV fluid rate
    C) Perform cervical examination

82. What characterizes a preterm fetal response to stress?
    A) Increased variability
    B) More frequently occurring variable decelerations
    C) More rapid deterioration from category I to II to III

83. Which factor influences blood flow to the uterus?
    A) Fetal arterial pressure
    B) Intervillous space flow
    C) Maternal arterial vasoconstriction

84. In a fetus with a single umbilical artery, what would the clinician expect to observe with Doppler flow studies?
    A) Decreased perfusion from the fetus to the placenta
    B) Decreased perfusion from the placenta to the fetus
    C) No change in blood flow between the fetus and the placenta

85. Betamethasone given to the pregnant patient can transiently affect the fetal heart rate (FHR) by:
    A) Decreasing variability
    B) Increasing variability
    C) Changing the baseline

86. A wandering fetal heart rate (FHR) baseline may be indicative of:
    A) Fetal seizure activity
    B) Impending fetal death
    C) Maternal medication administration

87. A fetal heart rate (FHR) pattern that is likely to be seen with maternal hypothermia is:
    A) Bradycardia
    B) Marked variability
    C) Tachycardia

88. The clinician supports the pregnant patient's decision to choose no extraordinary measures for a neonate who is about to deliver at 23 2/7 weeks' gestation. The clinician's support despite their own personal opinion is an example of:
    A) Autonomy
    B) Beneficence
    C) Justice

89. A preterm fetus has persistent supraventricular tachycardia (SVT) that is not hydropic. This is *best* treated by administering which drug to the pregnant patient?
    A) Amiodarone (Nexterone)
    B) Digoxin (Lanoxin)
    C) Flecainide (Tambocor)

90. Which of the following is the most likely cause of a prolonged deceleration?
    A) Chorioamnionitis
    B) Maternal hypertension
    C) Maternal hypotension

91. According to National Institute of Child Health and Human Development (NICHD) definitions, decelerations that occur with at least 50% of contractions are:
    A) Intermittent
    B) Recurrent
    C) Repetitive

92. Which medications used with preterm labor can affect fetal heart rate (FHR) characteristics?
    A) Antibiotics and narcotics
    B) Betamethasone and terbutaline
    C) Terbutaline and antibiotics

93. Following maternal position changes for recurrent variable decelerations, what is the *next* priority intervention?
    A) Amnioinfusion
    B) IV fluid bolus
    C) Preparation for Cesarean section

94. A modified biophysical profile (BPP) shows the following: Reactive nonstress test (NST) with moderate variability and maximum vertical pocket (MVP) of 2.6 cm. This test would be interpreted as:
    A) Abnormal
    B) Equivocal
    C) Normal

95. In a fetal heart rate (FHR) tracing with marked variability, which of the following is likely the cause?
    A) Fetal acidemia
    B) Recent ephedrine administration
    C) Recent epidural placement

96. As fetal hypoxia (asphyxia) worsens, the last component of the biophysical profile (BPP) to disappear is fetal:
    A) Breathing
    B) Movement
    C) Tone

97. Which of the following statements is *true* concerning the reliability of electronic fetal monitoring (EFM)?
    A) EFM has good interobserver reliability
    B) EFM has good intraobserver reliability
    C) EFM has poor interobserver and intraobserver reliability

98. Which of the following medications could be responsible for the following strip?

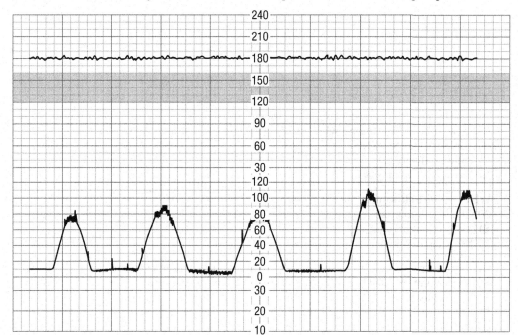

    A) Butorphanol
    B) Magnesium sulfate
    C) Terbutaline

99. A pregnant patient being monitored externally has a suspected placental abruption based on electronic fetal monitoring (EFM). The *most likely* type of deceleration noted is:
    A) Early
    B) Late
    C) Variable

100. Which of the following fetal heart characteristics can be determined using auscultation?
 A) Baseline rate
 B) Type of decelerations
 C) Variability

101. The clinician is evaluating a fetal heart rate (FHR) baseline. The finding that excludes the ability to determine the baseline is variability that is:
 A) Marked
 B) Minimal
 C) Moderate

102. While reviewing a pathology report after amniocentesis, which finding would the clinician understand to be indicative of a *decreased* risk for neonatal respiratory distress syndrome?
 A) Lecithin
 B) Phosphatidylglycerol
 C) Phosphorus

103. After applying an external monitor to a patient with premature rupture of membranes at 38 weeks' gestation, the clinician notes that the fetal heart rate (FHR) monitor is recording half the rate heard audibly. The clinician should:
 A) Apply a fetal scalp electrode
 B) Continue to monitor the patient
 C) Prepare the patient for an ultrasound

104. A patient receiving oxytocin (Pitocin) has 17 contractions in 30 minutes. According to National Institute of Child Health and Human Development (NICHD) guidelines, this is referred to as:
 A) Hyperstimulation
 B) Hypertonia
 C) Tachysystole

105. Administration of which of the following would be *least* likely to cause minimal variability in the term fetus?
 A) Ephedrine
 B) Magnesium sulfate
 C) Narcotics

106. When fetal lactic acid increases, there is a depletion in:
 A) Bicarbonate
 B) Carbonic acid
 C) Chloride

107. As fetal lactic acid increases, what is the impact on the fetal blood gas?
 A) Base deficit decreases
 B) Base deficit increases
 C) pH increases

108. Fetal blood is *most* oxygenated in the:
 A) Ductus arteriosus
 B) Ductus venosus
 C) Foramen ovale

109. A fetal heart rate (FHR) pattern that is associated with an abnormal acid-base status is:
 A) Minimal variability with no accelerations or decelerations
 B) Recurrent variable decelerations with moderate variability
 C) Tachycardia with absent variability

110. The supervising clinician notes that an orientee has repeatedly demonstrated competency interpreting basic fetal heart rate (FHR) patterns. The supervisor's next action is to:
    A) Develop comprehensive case studies for the orientee to review
    B) End the orientation process
    C) Periodically audit the orientee's patient medical records

111. Which of the following tachyarrhythmias can result in fetal hydrops?
    A) Persistent supraventricular tachycardia
    B) Premature atrial tachycardia
    C) Sinus tachycardia

112. A uterine rupture is typically suspected with the appearance of which fetal heart rate (FHR) pattern?
    A) Absent variability with intermittent late decelerations
    B) Minimal variability with variable decelerations
    C) Prolonged decelerations

113. Signal ambiguity occurs most frequently:
    A) During pushing when maternal heart rate rises more closely to fetal baseline
    B) When monitoring a multiple-gestation pregnancy
    C) With rupture of membranes

114. The greatest risk for fetal hypoxia is posed by maternal:
    A) Chronic disease
    B) Hypertension
    C) Hypotension

115. What would be a suspected pH in a fetus whose fetal heart tracing includes recurrent late decelerations during labor?
    A) 7.08
    B) 7.28
    C) 7.48

116. Which of the following describes the sequential progression of decompensation in the fetus when the oxygen pathway is interrupted?
    A) Hypoxemia, hypoxia, metabolic acidosis, and metabolic acidemia
    B) Hypoxia, hypoxemia, metabolic acidosis, and metabolic acidemia
    C) Metabolic acidemia, metabolic acidosis, hypoxia, and hypoxemia

117. The *minimum* expected response of the fetal heart rate (FHR) to active fetal movement in a fetus at a gestational age of 31 weeks is acceleration of at least:
    A) 10 beats per minute (bpm) for 10 seconds
    B) 10 bpm for 15 seconds
    C) 15 bpm for 10 seconds

118. When fetal chemoreceptors are activated, what happens to the fetal heart rate (FHR)?
    A) It decreases
    B) It increases
    C) It stays the same

119. The clinician is repositioning a laboring patient with a fetal scalp electrode in place. The recording of the fetal heart rate (FHR) pattern that the clinician may note on the tracing during repositioning is:
    A) Disorganized deflections of varying lengths
    B) Organized deflections at regular intervals of similar lengths
    C) Organized deflections of equal lengths

120. When the fetal baroreceptors are activated, the fetal heart rate (FHR):
    A) Decreases
    B) Increases
    C) Stays the same

121. A fetus with respiratory acidemia will have which of the following results?
A) pH 7.02, partial pressure of carbon dioxide (pCO_2) 66, bicarbonate (HCO_3) 24
B) pH 7.22, pCO_2 54, HCO_3 24
C) pH 7.02, pCO_2 54, HCO_3 18

122. What does the following strip most likely represent?

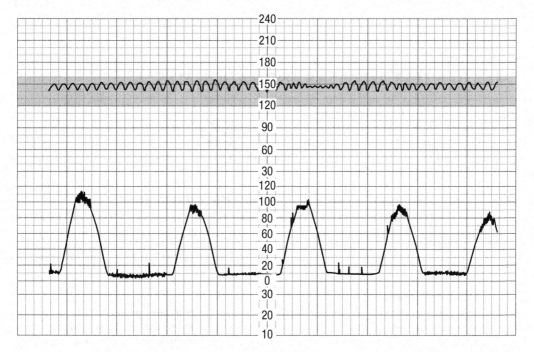

A) Active labor
B) Fetal anemia
C) Fetal intolerance of labor

123. The preterm fetus at 28 weeks' gestation will have minimal variability as a result of immaturity of which system?
A) Autonomic nervous
B) Endocrine
C) Respiratory

124. The nurse notes a pattern of decelerations on the fetal monitor, beginning shortly after the contraction and returning to baseline right before the contraction is over. The nurse's *best* response is to:
A) Give the patient oxygen by face mask at 8 to 10 L/min
B) Observe and record the pattern
C) Position the patient on the opposite side

125. A fetus with metabolic acidemia will have which of the following arterial blood gases?
A) pH 7.02, partial pressure of carbon dioxide (pCO_2) 66, bicarbonate (HCO_3) 24
B) pH 7.02, pCO_2 54, HCO_3 18
C) pH 7.22, pCO_2 54, HCO_3 24

10 Practice Test: Answers

Antay L. Waters

▶ PRACTICE TEST ANSWERS AND RATIONALES

1. B) FHR in relation to contractions
Fetal well-being is assessed during labor by evaluation of the FHR in relation to contractions. Evaluation of the FHR only does not give the clinician adequate information if decelerations are present. Evaluation of the uterine contraction pattern without the associated FHR does not provide any information related to fetal well-being.

2. B) EFM is a screening procedure that monitors FHR and contractions
EFM is a screening procedure that monitors both FHR and contractions. It is not a diagnostic procedure.

3. A) Aortic arch
Fetal chemoreceptors are located in the aortic arch. Fetal baroreceptors are located in the aortic arch and carotid bodies.

4. C) Variable decelerations
Variable decelerations are seen in the setting of oligohydramnios related to increased risk of cord compression due to lack of adequate amniotic fluid. Early decelerations are associated with fetal head compression, and late decelerations are seen in uteroplacental insufficiency. Early decelerations and late decelerations are not a risk inherent primarily to oligohydramnios.

5. C) Prepare for Cesarean section
The patient's presentation is highly suggestive of placental abruption, in which case an emergent Cesarean section is indicated. Terbutaline administration is contraindicated in the setting of placental abruption. Insertion of internal fetal monitors delays patient care and will provide no additional relevant clinical information.

6. B) Chemoreceptors
Chemoreceptors respond primarily to hypoxia and appear as late decelerations. Vagal responses are primarily characterized by bradycardia. Baroreceptors respond to changes in fetal blood pressure rather than to hypoxia.

7. A) 10-minute segment, excluding periodic or episodic changes
According to National Institute of Child Health and Human Development terminology, the baseline fetal heart rate is identified as an average rate of a 10-minute segment, excluding periodic or episodic changes.

8. C) Respiratory acidosis
Normal arterial pH in an uncomplicated delivery is greater than or equal to 7.10 for a term infant. The pH of 7.05 is consistent with acidosis. Normal arterial pO_2 is higher than 20, and normal pCO_2 is less than 60 mmHg; therefore, the infant has normal pO_2 and high pCO_2, which is consistent with respiratory acidosis. Base excess of more than –12 and base deficit of less than 12 are considered normal results.

9. A) Autonomy
Autonomy is the freedom of choice and the accepting of responsibility for one's choice. Autonomy means that the patient is able to make independent decisions. The concept of beneficence requires that actions taken be done to promote good and that clinicians act in the best interest of their patients. Justice requires that the distribution of benefits and burdens is equitable.

10. C) 7.02

Fetuses with a normal pH (>7) respond to scalp stimulation with an acceleration of the FHR. A fetus with a low pH of 6.92 or 6.95 would not respond to scalp stimulation with an acceleration of the FHR.

11. C) Help move the patient to a lateral position

It is reasonable to continue the oxytocin (Pitocin) and assist the patient to the lateral position to promote fetal oxygenation. An IV fluid bolus is not indicated. Discontinuing oxytocin (Pitocin) should not be the initial intervention in the case of a category I tracing.

12. C) 3 cm/min

EFM paper speed parameters in the United States are 3 cm/min for the horizontal axis and 30 beats per minute for the vertical axis.

13. C) Modified pushing

The initial resuscitative measure for a patient who is complete and pushing is to modify the pushing method. Neither amnioinfusion nor IV fluid bolus is indicated if the patient is complete and pushing because delivery is needed for resolution.

14. A) Making a recommendation

SBAR stands for **S**ituation, **B**ackground, **A**ssessment, **R**ecommendation. When using the SBAR communication tool, the "R" refers to making a recommendation. Reporting labs is part of the situation, and reviewing medical history is part of the background.

15. B) Heart rate

Unlike the adult heart, the fetal heart is not influenced by the Frank–Starling mechanism. The human fetal heart normally functions at the top of its cardiac function curve. Because the stroke volume does not fluctuate significantly, fetal cardiac output is essentially rate dependent. Fetal movement is not a contributing factor to cardiac output in early pregnancy.

16. B) Shunted toward the adrenal glands

During times of fetal stress, blood flow is shunted toward the heart, brain, and adrenal glands. It does not remain unchanged, and it is not shunted away from the adrenal glands.

17. C) 220 to 240

The most common fetal tachyarrhythmia is supraventricular tachycardia, which has absent-to-minimal variability and occurs at a rate of 220 to 240 bpm.

18. C) Variable decelerations with occasional late decelerations

Postterm pregnancies are at higher risk for uteroplacental insufficiency, leading to late decelerations, and oligohydramnios, leading to variable decelerations. While early decelerations may occur during the transitional phase of labor in the postterm pregnancy, they are not the most likely expectation. Marked variability is most often noted in response to a stressful intrapartum event that has not occurred frequently enough to cause overt acidemia.

19. C) Uteroplacental insufficiency

The tracing depicts late decelerations, which are associated with uteroplacental insufficiency. Early decelerations are associated with fetal head compression, and variable decelerations are associated with umbilical cord compression.

20. C) Vagus nerve

Maturation of the vagus nerve leads to a normal decline in the baseline fetal heart rate at approximately 26 to 28 weeks' gestation. Chemoreceptors respond primarily to hypoxia and appear as late decelerations. Baroreceptors respond to changes in fetal blood pressure rather than to hypoxia.

21. B) 110 to 160

The normal baseline fetal heart rate is 110 to 160 beats per minute. A range of 100 to 160 includes an abnormal baseline rate of 100 to 109 beats per minute, and a range of 120 to 160 excludes a normal baseline rate of 110 to 119 beats per minute.

22. C) They increase BP and decrease FHR
The increased catecholamines, along with increased blood flow to the heart, increase the fetal BP, while the FHR decreases secondary to oxygen deprivation.

23. C) 18
Significant neonatal morbidity is more likely to occur when more than 18 minutes elapses between the onset of significant fetal heart rate decelerations and delivery.

24. A) Intermittent
FHR decelerations that occur with less than 50% of contractions are termed *intermittent*, whereas those that occur with greater than 50% of contractions are referred to as *recurrent*. "Repetitive" is not a term that is part of the NICHD terminology for FHR characteristics.

25. B) Insert a fetal spiral electrode and turn off the logic
To adequately monitor and evaluate a suspected fetal arrhythmia, a spiral fetal scalp electrode must be placed and the logic turned off. While external monitoring or Doppler may be used, they are not the most accurate methods for monitoring and evaluation.

26. C) Recurrent late decelerations with minimal variability
A category III fetal tracing is characterized by a sinusoidal pattern *or* by recurrent late decelerations with absent variability. Recurrent late decelerations with minimal variability is considered a category II fetal tracing.

27. B) Performing a cervical exam
Performing a cervical exam allows for simultaneous fetal scalp stimulation. Providing juice to the patient and initiating maternal position changes may elicit an acceleration but would not be as timely and thus are not the best options.

28. A) Baseline change
A fetal heart rate change lasting for at least 10 minutes is termed a baseline change rather than a deceleration. At 110 bpm, the fetal heart rate is still within normal limits. A prolonged deceleration lasts anywhere between 2 and 10 minutes.

29. C) Category III
A smooth, undulating wave pattern without variability is a sinusoidal pattern. By National Institute of Child Health and Human Development definitions, a sinusoidal pattern is a category III fetal tracing.

30. B) Late
Late decelerations are the result of decreased oxygenation, often secondary to placental insufficiency. Variable decelerations are most often related to cord compression, whereas early decelerations are most often related to fetal head compression.

31. C) 3, 2, 1
When a fetal tracing appears to be sinusoidal, the first step is to determine if it is true sinusoidal versus only sinusoidal appearing from recent narcotic administration. Following this determination, the patient should be placed in either right or left lateral position. Finally, if unresolved, the clinician should prepare for Cesarean delivery.

32. C) Notify the attending physician or midwife
Notification of the physician or midwife is the appropriate response to this situation because variability cannot be determined via auscultation, and application of a fetal scalp electrode is contraindicated in a patient with HIV.

33. C) Vagal stimulation
Stimulation of the fetal vagus nerve during maternal pushing efforts may result in fetal bradycardia. Fetal hypoxemia would result in decreased variability or increased fetal heart rate. Fetal rotation does not inherently lead to bradycardia.

34. C) Uteroplacental insufficiency

Late decelerations are the result of decreased oxygenation, often secondary to placental insufficiency. Variable decelerations are most often related to cord compression, while early decelerations are most often related to fetal head compression.

35. C) 15 bpm for at least 15 seconds

According to National Institute of Child Health and Human Development definitions, an acceleration of the fetal heart rate after 32 weeks' gestation is defined as a rise in the FHR of at least 15 bpm for at least 15 seconds. Prior to 32 weeks, an acceleration is the rise of the FHR for at least 10 bpm for at least 10 seconds.

36. B) Loss of variability with recurrent late or variable decelerations

Progressive fetal hypoxia is characterized by increasing loss of variability with recurrent nonreassuring decelerations. Moderate variability is not present in the setting of fetal hypoxia.

37. A) Fetal heart block

Fetal autoimmune atrioventricular (AV) block is typically seen in association with autoimmune antibodies in the pregnant patient that cross the placenta and damage the fetal AV node. These antibodies would not lead to premature ventricular contraction or fetal supraventricular tachycardia because damage to the AV node leads to a lower fetal heart rate.

38. B) .9% sodium chloride

.9% sodium chloride, or normal saline, is one of two appropriate IV fluids for amnioinfusion; the other one is lactated Ringer's solution. Half normal saline and dextrose 5% in normal saline are not appropriate IV fluids for intrauterine resuscitation.

39. A) Fetal heart block

Fetal heart block leads to fetal bradycardia, not fetal tachycardia. Both maternal fever and sympathomimetic drugs, such as epinephrine (Adrenalin) or norepinephrine (Levophed), lead to fetal tachycardia.

40. B) Moderate variability

The aspect of electronic fetal monitoring most predictive of a well-oxygenated fetus is moderate variability. A stable baseline rate and absence of decelerations may be reassuring overall but could lack the variability associated with a well-oxygenated fetus.

41. A) Brain

During a hypoxic episode, fetal blood is shunted to the fetal brain because the fetal liver and lungs are not life-sustaining while the fetus is in utero.

42. A) Continue providing care to the patient and write a late entry after the Cesarean section is complete

Continuing to provide care to the patient and writing a late entry after the emergent Cesarean section is the most appropriate approach. It is not appropriate to ask someone else, including the charge nurse, to write an entry in the electronic health record about a conversation they were not a part of. Patient care should never be sacrificed for documentation purposes.

43. C) Maternal fever in the presence of fetal tachycardia does not necessarily require Cesarean delivery

The clinical picture is consistent with chorioamnionitis secondary to prolonged rupture of membranes. Maternal fever in the presence of fetal tachycardia does not necessarily require Cesarean section because the patient is making good labor progress and is in active labor. Fetal heart failure occurs with sustained fetal tachycardia over days to weeks, not hours. There is no imminent danger of fetal heart failure related to fetal tachycardia. Cesarean section does not prevent the development of fetal sepsis.

44. B) Maternal repositioning

The initial intervention for recurrent late decelerations with preserved variability should be maternal repositioning. Amnioinfusion has no impact on late decelerations. While oxygen is an option, it is no longer supported by evidence, and initial treatment should include maternal position changes. Per the American College of Obstetricians and Gynecologists, the routine use of oxygen supplementation with normal oxygen saturation is not recommended for fetal intrauterine resuscitation.

45. B) Fetal hemoglobin is higher than adult hemoglobin

Fetal hemoglobin is higher than adult hemoglobin. Fetal hemoglobin has a *higher* affinity for oxygen than adult hemoglobin. When there is an abrupt decrease in oxygen, the fetus compensates by redistributing blood to the brain, heart, and adrenal glands—*not* to the lungs.

46. B) Fetal congestive heart failure

Sustained, prolonged fetal SVT may lead to fetal congestive heart failure, but not to fetal heart block, as this occurs below the level at which fetal SVT originates. Fetal SVT has no bearing on maternal cardiac status.

47. C) Variability and accelerations

While the fetal heart rate provides valuable information, variability and accelerations are the two most reassuring components of fetal monitoring.

48. C) Varied in depth and duration

Oligohydramnios often results in variable decelerations, which can be described as varied in depth and duration. Decelerations that are late in onset or occur after the peak of the contraction are late decelerations, whereas those that are synchronous with the contraction are early decelerations—neither of which are directly associated with oligohydramnios.

49. B) Kidneys

The fetal kidneys have the greatest influence on fetal pH because they are able to reabsorb filtered bicarbonate and generate new bicarbonate. The fetal heart and nervous system are not actively involved in fetal acid-base metabolism.

50. C) Acceleration

Fetal scalp stimulation of a well-oxygenated fetus should elicit an acceleration, not a deceleration or a baseline change.

51. B) Comparing maternal pulse with fetal heart rate

The first step in assessing a low fetal heart rate is ensuring that the maternal heart rate is not being traced instead of the fetal heart rate. The next steps involve placing external monitors, removing the fetal scalp electrode, and notifying the provider.

52. C) Resting tone less than 20 to 25 mmHg

Normal uterine resting tone is 20 to 25 mmHg. Contractions occurring every 1 to 2 minutes is considered uterine tachysystole. Uterine contractions with an intensity of 100 mmHg in early labor are outside the normal range of 25 to 75 mmHg.

53. A) Decreasing

In a patient admitted with preeclampsia with severe features, routine management necessitates the use of magnesium sulfate, which decreases fetal heart rate variability.

54. A) Early

Early decelerations are characteristic of fetal head compression, which can be seen in cephalopelvic disproportion, particularly in early labor. Late decelerations are characteristic of hypoxia and uteroplacental insufficiency, while variable decelerations are characteristic of cord compression.

55. A) 10

Baseline fetal heart rate is determined over a 10-minute period. Any change in the fetal heart rate lasting more than 10 minutes is considered a baseline change.

56. A) Butorphanol
Butorphanol is known to cause sinusoidal-appearing fetal heart rate patterns that are not seen with morphine and fentanyl administration.

57. A) 5 minutes
The accepted monitoring interval for low-risk patients in second stage labor is every 5 minutes according to the most recent recommendations by American College of Obstetricians and Gynecologists and American Academy of Pediatrics Joint Guidelines and by the American College of Nurse-Midwives.

58. B) Cervical examination
In a patient with a prolonged deceleration immediate after spontaneous rupture of membranes, umbilical cord prolapse must be excluded by cervical exam. While maternal position changes may be initiated after discovery of a prolapsed cord, a cervical exam must be performed first. Amnioinfusion is not indicated for a prolonged deceleration.

59. B) Late
Late decelerations are considered neurogenic in origin and are frequently amenable to intrauterine resuscitation techniques aimed at maximizing uterine blood flow, often in the setting of uteroplacental insufficiency. The decrease in fetal partial pressure of oxygen (pO_2) leads to an autonomic fetal response causing intense vasoconstriction. Baroreceptors perceive the increase in blood pressure; ultimately, stimulating a parasympathetic response causes a late deceleration. Variable declarations are most often related to umbilical cord compression through activation of the baroreceptors in the aortic arch and internal carotid arteries. Early decelerations are always in association with contractions and are suggested to be the result of a nonhypoxic reflex secondary to increased intracranial pressure. While also neurogenic in origin, early decelerations are not amenable to intrauterine resuscitation.

60. C) Variable
Monoamniotic-monochorionic twins are most prone to variable decelerations during labor secondary to cord entanglement. Cord entanglement does not lead to early or late decelerations.

61. C) Discontinuing the oxytocin (Pitocin)
The first action in a patient with oxytocin-induced tachysystole with indeterminate EFM tracing is discontinuation of oxytocin (Pitocin). Removal of this offending factor may resolve the tachycardia. While IV fluids and maternal position changes may provide some assistance, oxytocin (Pitocin) discontinuation is required in a patient with oxytocin-induced tachysystole with an indeterminate EFM tracing.

62. B) Intrauterine pressure catheter
The most sensitive method for uterine activity assessment is an intrauterine pressure catheter. An external tocotransducer does not provide the same level of accuracy and can be limited by maternal body habitus. Manual palpation is subjective by examiner.

63. B) Umbilical cord compression
Variable decelerations are most often related to cord compression, while early decelerations are most often related to fetal head compression. Late decelerations are the result of decreased oxygenation, often secondary to placental insufficiency.

64. C) Multifetal gestation
Multifetal gestation pregnancies are more prone to variable decelerations. Maternal diabetes mellitus and collagen vascular disease are common causes for late decelerations related to their impact on the placenta.

65. C) Maternal position changes
The first action for variable decelerations should be maternal position changes. For recurrent variable decelerations, an amnioinfusion and/or maternal oxygen administration may be considered if maternal oxygen saturation is low.

66. A) External tocodynamometer

Resting tone and intensity may be accurately assessed via manual palpation, although this may vary by clinician and intrauterine pressure catheter. It cannot be accurately assessed by external tocodynamometer because this is useful only for determining approximate contraction frequency and duration as well as relative changes.

67. C) Administer terbutaline (Brethine)

Given the uterine contraction frequency and the prolonged fetal heart rate deceleration, the next action should be terbutaline (Brethine) administration to decrease contraction frequency and allow the fetus to recover. Administration of $MgSO_4$ or IV fluid bolus will not decrease the frequency of contractions in an efficient manner to allow for fetal recovery.

68. C) Performing fetal scalp stimulation

Fetal scalp stimulation is contraindicated during a prolonged deceleration, whereas assisting the patient to right lateral position may improve fetal oxygenation status. Performing a cervical exam is indicated to rule out cord prolapse.

69. A) Decreases

When the fetal parasympathetic nervous system is stimulated, the fetal heart rate decreases, whereas stimulation of the sympathetic nervous system causes the fetal heart rate to increase.

70. B) Decrease in variability

Administration of betamethasone for fetal lung maturity as well as magnesium sulfate for preterm labor and fetal neuroprotection may cause a decrease in the fetal heart rate variability without having an impact on the fetal heart rate baseline.

71. B) Increased baseline and variable decelerations

A preterm fetus typically has a higher baseline related to the immature parasympathetic nervous system. Due to sympathetic dominance, the preterm fetus also tends to have less variability. Variable decelerations in the preterm fetus are believed to be related to the smaller amount of Wharton's jelly in the umbilical cord to protect from cord compression seen in variable decelerations. Accelerations are transient in the preterm fetus.

72. A) Low-amplitude, high-frequency contractions

Low-amplitude, high-frequency contractions are often noted in preterm labor and may lead to cervical change. Uterine irritability may be seen throughout pregnancy and does not lead to cervical change. Tetanic contractions are often indicative of a more serious condition, such as placental abruption.

73. C) Not changed

Despite the widespread use of electronic fetal monitoring, the rate of cerebral palsy has remained the same.

74. B) Higher

In comparison with maternal blood, fetal blood has a higher affinity for oxygen.

75. C) Variable

Variable decelerations are the most frequently encountered fetal heart rate abnormality, particularly because they are common in preterm fetuses, and many occur throughout pregnancy secondary to umbilical cord compression.

76. C) Hypothyroidism

Maternal hypothyroidism does not lead to fetal tachycardia, whereas maternal fever and maternal hyperthyroidism may both lead to fetal tachycardia.

77. A) Breech presentation

Breech presentation is not an indication for antepartum fetal testing; however, both gestational hypertension and gestational diabetes are indications for antepartum fetal testing due to risk for fetal distress and adverse outcomes.

78. A) Active transport
Active transport is used for the transfer of amino acids, water-soluble vitamins, calcium, phosphorus, iron, and iodine across the placenta. Oxygen, carbon dioxide, sodium, chloride, and glucose cross the placenta by passive diffusion. Water moves by simple diffusion according to hydrostatic and osmotic pressure gradients.

79. A) Back
Placement of the ultrasound transducer over the fetal back yields the best EFM recording. Placement over the fetal chest may yield distant or muffled sounds with more potential for discontinuous tracing. Placement over the fetal abdomen, or stomach, may yield either inaudible or very muffled fetal heart tones.

80. A) Early
During the transitional phase of labor, early decelerations are common because fetal head compression occurs during descent. Although variable decelerations may be seen during the second stage, they are less likely during the transitional phase. Late decelerations are the result of uteroplacental insufficiency and are not directly associated with the transitional phase of labor.

81. C) Perform cervical examination
Performing a cervical examination simply to assess fetal tachycardia increases the risk of chorioamnionitis and does not provide additional information. Increasing maternal IV fluids may decrease fetal tachycardia. Assessment of maternal vital signs could reveal maternal fever as a potential cause of fetal tachycardia.

82. C) More rapid deterioration from category I to II to III
The preterm fetus is more likely to be subjected to and affected by hypoxia than the term fetus, leading to a more rapid progression to a category III electronic fetal monitoring tracing. Stress does not lead to variable decelerations and may cause decreased, not increased, variability.

83. C) Maternal arterial vasoconstriction
Maternal arterial vasoconstriction influences blood flow through the placenta to the uterus. Higher vasoconstriction decreases uterine blood flow. The flow within the intervillous space does not directly affect blood flow to the uterus. Fetal arterial pressure also does not impact blood flow to the uterus, only maternal factors.

84. A) Decreased perfusion from the fetus to the placenta
Because there are normally two umbilical arteries flowing from the fetus to the placenta, the absence of one of these will lead to decreased blood perfusion from the fetus to the placenta. There is no impact on perfusion from the placenta to the fetus because this flow occurs through the umbilical vein.

85. A) Decreasing variability
Administration of betamethasone for fetal lung maturity may cause a decrease in the fetal heart rate variability without an impact on the fetal heart rate baseline.

86. B) Impending fetal death
A wandering FHR baseline is most often indicative of impending fetal death in a neurologically abnormal fetus. Maternal medication administration may impact variability, but it does not cause a wandering baseline. Fetal seizures would be more likely to appear on electronic fetal monitoring as a hypoxic episode, such as late decelerations, but it should be confirmed by ultrasound.

87. A) Bradycardia
Just as a maternal fever may lead to fetal tachycardia, maternal hypothermia may produce fetal bradycardia; however, moderate variability is maintained because the pattern is not indicative of fetal hypoxia.

88. A) Autonomy
Autonomy is respecting the patient's (or parent's) right to choose and exercise their personal opinions. Beneficence requires that the actions taken be done in the best interest of the patient. Justice requires the equitable distribution of benefits and burden.

89. B) Digoxin (Lanoxin)

In nonhydropic fetuses with SVT, digoxin (Lanoxin) therapy is recommended. Flecainide (Tambocor) and amiodarone (Nexterone) are reserved for hydropic fetuses with SVT because digoxin (Lanoxin) may be ineffective in these cases.

90. C) Maternal hypotension

Maternal hypotension, such as occurs immediately after regional anesthesia or major trauma, may lead to a prolonged deceleration due to placental blood flow being insufficient to maintain the fetal heart rate at a normal level. Chorioamnionitis is more likely to cause fetal tachycardia. Maternal hypertension is more likely to lead to late decelerations related to intermittent uteroplacental insufficiency.

91. B) Recurrent

Decelerations that occur with at least 50% of contractions are recurrent. Decelerations that occur with less than 50% of contractions are intermittent. "Repetitive" is not a term that is part of the NICHD accepted terminology.

92. B) Betamethasone and terbutaline

Betamethasone and narcotics may decrease variability. Terbutaline may increase the fetal heart rate baseline. Antibiotics have no effect on fetal heart rate characteristics.

93. A) Amnioinfusion

Amnioinfusion is the next priority intervention for recurrent variable decelerations, following maternal position changes. While an IV fluid bolus may be initiated, it does not have an immediate impact. Preparation for Cesarean section should occur only in the setting of fetal distress associated with variable decelerations that are not resolved with maternal position changes and amnioinfusion.

94. C) Normal

A modified BPP with a reactive NST and moderate variability with normal amniotic fluid index is a normal test. If either the NST were nonreactive or the MVP were less than 2 cm, the test would be abnormal. There is no equivocal result in a modified BPP.

95. A) Fetal acidemia

Fetal acidemia may cause marked variability due to an increased sympathetic response secondary to a stressful intrapartum event (cord compression, meconium) and increased lactate level, but it does not necessarily increase risk of neonatal mortality. Maternal ephedrine administration is associated with significant increases in fetal heart rate and beat-to-beat variability. Recent epidural placement is more likely to cause maternal hypotension leading to prolonged decelerations.

96. C) Tone

In the continuum of fetal distress of acidosis, hypoxia, and asphyxia, fetal breathing movements are lost first, followed by body movements, with extremity tone being the final component lost.

97. C) EFM has poor interobserver and intraobserver reliability

Despite recent efforts to increase education related to EFM interpretation, poor interobserver and intraobserver reliability remain. The implementation of additional training and certification programs is aimed at improving these statistics.

98. C) Terbutaline

Terbutaline may lead to intermittent, self-terminating fetal tachycardia as shown in the tracing. Magnesium sulfate administration is associated with decreased variability. Butorphanol administration is associated with a sinusoidal-appearing pattern.

99. B) Late

Prior to becoming terminal bradycardic, a patient with a placental abruption will most likely have late decelerations due to the interruption of placental blood flow. Variable declarations are associated with umbilical cord compression, whereas early decelerations are associated with fetal head compression, neither of which are seen in placental abruption.

100. A) Baseline rate
Auscultation may be used to determine baseline rate and presence or absence of accelerations and decelerations. Variability and type of deceleration cannot be determined with auscultation.

101. A) Marked
The significance of a fetal heart rate with marked variability and a pronounced beat-to-beat range is uncertain and prevents the accurate interpretation of the baseline rate. Moderate variability is associated with autonomic regulation of the fetal heart rate not affected by any interruption in oxygenation. Minimal variability can be associated with fetal metabolic acidemia, preexisting neurologic injuries, or fetal sleep cycles.

102. B) Phosphatidylglycerol
Phosphatidylglycerol is the glycerophospholipid found in pulmonary surfactant and is a precursor to surfactant. Its presence is indicative of fetal lung maturity and decreased risk for neonatal respiratory distress syndrome. Phosphorous is not a substance associated with respiratory distress syndrome. Lecithin is measured in conjunction with another phospholipid, sphingomyelin, in a ratio to assess fetal lung maturity.

103. A) Apply a fetal scalp electrode
Fetal dysrhythmias can only be recorded using a fetal EKG; therefore, a fetal scalp electrode will need to be applied for confirmation. An external monitor will not provide the clinician with a continuous tracing. An ultrasound allows for visual assessment of the fetal heart but does not provide a continuous tracing.

104. C) Tachysystole
Tachysystole is the NICHD term for more than 15 contractions during a 30-minute period. *Hyperstimulation* and *hypertonia* are not part of NICHD terminology.

105. A) Ephedrine
Ephedrine administration is more likely to cause fetal tachycardia and increased variability, whereas magnesium sulfate or narcotics administration is more likely to cause minimal variability.

106. A) Bicarbonate
When fetal lactic acid increases, fetal partial pressure of carbon dioxide and bicarbonate levels are decreased. Chloride and carbonic acid levels are unaffected.

107. B) Base deficit increases
As fetal lactic acid levels increase, the base deficit increases and the pH decreases.

108. B) Ductus venosus
Fetal blood is most oxygenated in the ductus venosus, which allows highly oxygenated blood to bypass the liver to the inferior vena cava then to the right atrium. The patent foramen ovale allows oxygen-rich blood to move from the right to the left atrium and mix with less oxygenated blood. The ductus arteriosus sends oxygen-poor blood back through the umbilical arteries to the placenta to pick up oxygen.

109. C) Tachycardia with absent variability
Variability is the best predictor of fetal oxygenation and acid-base balance. Absent variability is most likely indicative of abnormal acid-base status, regardless of the presence of variable decelerations.

110. A) Develop comprehensive case studies for the orientee to review
Developing comprehensive case studies will assist the orientee in evaluating situations beyond simple interpretations and will better prepare the orientee to provide safe care to patients. Taking the orientee off orientation or periodically auditing patient medical records will not offer the opportunity for growth related to fetal heart rate interpretation.

111. A) Persistent supraventricular tachycardia
Untreated persistent supraventricular tachycardia may result in fetal hydrops. Premature atrial tachycardia and sinus tachycardia are generally considered benign.

112. C) Prolonged decelerations
Uterine rupture is typically associated with terminal bradycardia, prolonged decelerations, or recurrent late decelerations, not variable or intermittent late decelerations.

113. A) During pushing when maternal heart rate rises more closely to fetal baseline
Signal ambiguity can be seen when the maternal heart rate becomes tachycardic with the work of pushing. If there is an acceleration with pushing, the maternal heart rate should be suspected because the fetus is more likely to have a deceleration due to a vagal response.

114. C) Hypotension
Maternal hypotension poses the greatest risk for fetal hypoxia because of decreased placental perfusion of oxygenated blood. Maternal hypertension increases the risk for placental abruption and uteroplacental insufficiency. Maternal chronic diseases pose a variety of fetal risks; however, as a whole, they do not pose the greatest risk for fetal hypoxia.

115. A) 7.08
Recurrent late decelerations are often indicative of fetal acidemia. Normal umbilical cord gas pH is greater than or equal to 7.10.

116. C) Metabolic acidemia, metabolic acidosis, hypoxia, and hypoxemia
Fetal decompensation secondary to interruption in normal oxygen pathways progresses from metabolic acidemia to metabolic acidosis to hypoxia to hypoxemia.

117. A) 10 beats per minute (bpm) for 10 seconds
According to National Institute of Child Health and Human Development definitions, an acceleration of the fetal heart rate prior to 32 weeks' gestation is expected to be a rise of at least 10 bpm for at least 10 seconds. While a greater increase for a longer period of time is acceptable and reassuring, the minimum is 10 bpm for at least 10 seconds. After 32 weeks' gestation, an acceleration is defined as a rise in the fetal heart rate of at least 15 bpm for at least 15 seconds.

118. A) It decreases
The fetal heart rate decreases through the interaction of the central and peripheral chemoreceptors. Activation of chemoreceptors may result in late decelerations, variable decelerations, and prolonged decelerations.

119. A) Disorganized deflections of varying lengths
Artifact can occur when the connection points of the monitor are disrupted, such as during maternal movement. It is characterized by disorganized deflections of varying lengths. Dysrhythmias are characterized by organized deflections of equal lengths or organized deflections at regular intervals of similar lengths, which would not be seen when repositioning a patient.

120. A) Decreases
The fetal heart rate decreases due to activation of baroreceptors via stretching, sending signals to the vagus nerve. Activation of baroreceptors may result in variable and prolonged decelerations.

121. A) pH 7.02, partial pressure of carbon dioxide (pCO$_2$) 66, bicarbonate (HCO$_3$) 24
A fetus with respiratory acidemia will have decreased pH, increased carbon dioxide, and normal HCO$_3$. Results of pH 7.02, pCO$_2$ 66, and HCO$_3$ 24 are consistent with respiratory acidemia. pH 7.22, pCO$_2$ 54, and HCO$_3$ 24 represent a normal umbilical cord gas. pH 7.02, pCO$_2$ 54, and HCO$_3$ 18 are consistent with metabolic acidemia.

122. B) Fetal anemia
A true sinusoidal pattern is most often the result of fetal anemia. Neither active labor nor fetal intolerance of labor will lead to a true sinusoidal pattern.

123. A) Autonomic nervous

The preterm fetus will have minimal variability and a higher baseline heart rate related to an immature autonomic nervous system. While the fetus also has immature endocrine and respiratory systems, these systems do not affect the fetal heart rate.

124. B) Observe and record the pattern

This pattern of deceleration is an early deceleration and requires no intervention; early deceleration is reassuring in normal labor. Repositioning is indicated for variable and late decelerations. Oxygen is indicated when maternal oxygen saturation is low.

125. B) pH 7.02, pCO$_2$ 54, HCO$_3$ 18

A fetus with metabolic acidemia will have decreased pH, normal carbon dioxide, and decreased HCO$_3$. pH of 7.02, pCO$_2$ of 66, and HCO$_3$ of 24 are consistent with respiratory acidemia. pH of 7.22, pCO$_2$ of 54, and HCO$_3$ of 24 indicate a normal umbilical cord gas.

Index